THE COMPLETE MRCPsych
PART I

THE COMPLETE MRCPsych
PART I

A comprehensive guide to the examination

Edited by Ashok G Patel MBBS, DPM, FRCPsych
Consultant in General Adult Psychiatry
Bedford Hospital
Bedford, UK

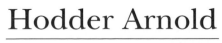

Hodder Arnold

A MEMBER OF THE HODDER HEADLINE GROUP

First published in Great Britain in 2006 by
Hodder Arnold, an imprint of
Hodder Education and a member of the Hodder Headline Group,
338 Euston Road, London NW1 3BH

http://www.hoddereducation.com

Distributed in the United States of America by
Oxford University Press Inc.,
198 Madison Avenue, New York, NY10016
Oxford is a registered trademark of Oxford University Press

Whilst the advice and information in this book are believed to be true and accurate at the date of
going to press, neither the author[s] nor the publisher can accept any legal responsibility or
liability for any errors or omissions that may be made. In particular, (but without limiting the
generality of the preceding disclaimer) every effort has been made to check drug dosages; however
it is still possible that errors have been missed. Furthermore, dosage schedules are constantly being
revised and new side-effects recognized. For these reasons the reader is strongly urged to consult
the drug companies' printed instructions before administering any of the drugs recommended in
this book.

British Library Cataloguing in Publication Data
A catalogue record for this book is available from the British Library

Library of Congress Cataloging-in-Publication Data
A catalog record for this book is available from the Library of Congress

ISBN-10   0 340 90811 4
ISBN-13   978 0 340 90811 2

1 2 3 4 5 6 7 8 9 10

Commissioning Editor: Clare Christian
Project Editor: Clare Patterson
Production Controller: Jane Lawrence
Cover Design: Nichola Smith
Index: Laurence Errington

Typeset in 9.5 on 12pt Rotis serif by Phoenix Photosetting, Chatham, Kent
Printed and bound in Malta.

What do you think about this book? Or any other Hodder Arnold title?
Please send your comments to www.hoddereducation.com

CONTENTS

List of contributors   vii
Foreword   ix
Preface   xi

Section 1: A Guide to the MRCPsych Part I Examination

1 Format of the MRCPsych Part I examination   *Ashok G Patel*   3
2 Outline of the written paper   *Ashok G Patel*   5
3 Outline of the curriculum   *Ashok G Patel*   6
4 ISQs and EMIs and how to tackle them   *Ashok G Patel*   9
5 Explanation of terms used in ISQ and EMI papers   *Kirti Singh*   12
6 OSCEs: aims, advantages and disadvantages   *Ashok G Patel*   13
7 Skills to be tested in OSCEs   *Ashok G Patel*   16
8 Format of OSCEs   *Simmi Sachdeva-Mohan*   17
9 Marking of OSCEs   *Ashok G Patel*   18
10 Preparing for OSCEs   *Ashok G Patel*   19
11 How to tackle OSCEs   *Ashok G Patel*   23

Section 2: Papers

1 Paper 1 (ISQs)
     Questions   *Kirti Singh and Ashok G Patel*   29
     Answers and explanations   *Kirti Singh and Ashok G Patel*   43
2 Paper 2 (ISQs)
     Questions   *Vishelle Ramkisson and Sanjith Kamath*   52
     Answers and explanations   *Sanjith Kamath and Vishelle Ramkisson*   66
3 Paper 3 (ISQs)
     Questions   *Ashok G Patel and Kirti Singh*   75
     Answers and explanations   *Ashok G Patel and Kirti Singh*   89
4 Paper 4 (ISQs)
     Questions   *Ashok G Patel*   99
     Answers and explanations   *Ashok G Patel*   113
5 Paper 5 (ISQs)
     Questions   *Kallol Sain and Milind Karale*   123
     Answers and explanations   *Milind Karale and Kallol Sain*   137
6 Paper 6 (ISQs)
     Questions   *Ashok G Patel and Elizabeth Barron*   148
     Answers and explanations   *Elizabeth Barron and Ashok G Patel*   162
7 Paper 7 (EMIs)
     Questions   *Ajay Upadhyaya and Ashok G Patel*   171
     Answers   *Ashok G Patel and Ajay Upadhyaya*   221

Further reading   *Simmi Sachdeva-Mohan and Ashok G Patel*   229
Index   233

CONTRIBUTORS

Ashok G Patel MBBS DPM FRCPsych
Consultant in General Adult Psychiatry
Bedford Hospital
Bedford
UK

Elizabeth Barron MBChB MRCPsych
Specialist Registrar
Bedford Hospital
Bedford
UK

Sanjith Kamath MBBS, MRCPsych
Specialist Registrar
Broadfields Hospital
Cambridge
UK

Milind Karale MBBS, DPM, DNB, MRCPsych
Specialist Registrar
Fulbourn Hospital
Cambridge
UK

Vishelle Ramkisson MBBS, MRCPsych
Specialist Registrar
Peterborough District Hospital
Peterborough
UK

Simmi Sachdeva-Mohan MBBS, DPM, MD, MRCPsych
Specialist Registrar
Rampton Hospital
Nottingham
UK

Kallol Sain MBBS, DPM, MRCPsych
Specialist Registrar
Fulbourn Hospital
Cambridge
UK

Kirti Singh MBBS, PGDLMS
Senior House Officer in Accident and Emergency Medicine
Luton and Dunstable Hospital
Luton
UK

Ajay Upadhyaya DPM, MD, FRCP (Canada), FRCPsych
Consultant Psychiatrist
Herts and Essex Hospital
Bishop's Stortford
UK

FOREWORD

Dr Ashok G Patel has an impressive track record of commitment to ensuring quality in psychiatric training and to championing the interests of trainees. Working with him in the years that I was Dean of the Royal College of Psychiatrists was a privilege and a pleasure.

In this book Dr Patel and the team of co-authors he has marshalled provide a comprehensive guide to the Part I MRCPsych examination which reflects the depth of his understanding of the trainee's position. As well as providing a guide to the curriculum and a comprehensive range of questions in all the formats used in the examination, the book provides explanations for the answers, suggested background reading and, most important, a detailed historical background and rationale for why the exam now takes the form it does.

Trainees need all appropriate help and support in preparing to take their examinations. This book is an important aid both to them and to their supervisors in ensuring that they supplement their knowledge, skills and attitudes with focused exam practice. I congratulate Dr Patel for having brought this project to fruition and wish success to all trainees who use the book!

Professor Cornelius Katona
Former Dean, Royal College of Psychiatrists

PREFACE

This book is the product of many years' experience of clinical psychiatry and teaching both under- and postgraduate students in psychiatry. It should serve as a framework to prepare for all topics of the different components of the MRCPsych Part I examination. It should also serve as a tool to test the knowledge of candidates taking this examination. The book is primarily aimed at senior house officers and other doctors (both referred to as candidates throughout the book). However, college tutors, coordinating tutors, specialist registrars and consultant psychiatrists/educational supervisors will also find it helpful in teaching and training their colleagues for the examination. I believe that the book will allow readers to become familiar with both the format and contents of the examination leading to success in the actual examination.

As the title of the book suggests, I have tried to cover all aspects of the curriculum for the examination. The book contains six papers of Individual Statement Questions (ISQs) with answers and explanations where necessary, one paper of Extended Matching Items (EMIs) questions with answers and a section on all aspects of Objective Structured Clinical Examinations (OSCEs). More importantly, guidance is provided on how to prepare for the examination, i.e. from the time of decision to take the examination until the day of taking it, and how to tackle it on the actual day. The ISQs papers contain a range of questions arranged under headings in the manner they appear in the examination. Candidates will therefore be able to concentrate their minds better, rather than when going through questions that are arranged randomly.

Throughout the book, my purpose has been to provide sufficient information for each component of the curriculum rather than a full account. It is therefore assumed that candidates will read textbooks and other publications before and while attempting the sample questions for obtaining more information. I have tried my best to give accurate answers and explanations to the ISQs and answers to EMIs. However, it is possible that inaccuracy may have crept into the book. I would therefore advise readers to refer to textbooks and other authentic sources of information to verify the answers if necessary.

The Further Reading section includes a carefully selected list of books and other publications following advice from college tutors and trainees who passed their examination in recent years. As this is meant to be a guide to the examination, references for every statement are not provided. The candidates are advised to refer to the Further Reading section and other sources for relevant references if required.

I would like to thank the other contributors who volunteered to participate in production of this book. I would like to thank the trainees who helped me to peer review the ISQs and EMIs and hopefully improve their quality. My sincere thanks to Professor Cornelius Katona for his most helpful encouragement, advice and generosity in providing a Foreword. I am most grateful to the staff of Hodder Arnold, especially Clare Christian, Clare Patterson and Lotika Singha for their advice and support throughout the preparation of the book.

It would not have been possible to produce this work without the support of our families.

A G P

SECTION 1:
A GUIDE TO THE MRCPsych PART I EXAMINATION

1 FORMAT OF THE MRCPsych PART I EXAMINATION

Written examination

The MRCPsych Part I written paper consists of:

* 133 Individual Statement Questions (ISQs)
* 30 Extended Matching Items (EMIs)

The EMIs are based on 10 themes. Each EMI has four components: the theme, options, lead-in (i.e. instructions) and three questions.

Time

The allotted time for the written paper is 90 minutes. Candidates are advised to spend approximately 60 minutes on the ISQs and 30 minutes on the EMIs.

Marking system

There are a total of 223 marks for the written paper. Of these, 133 marks are for the ISQs and 90 marks are for the EMIs. Each candidate's marks in the ISQ and EMI sections are combined and converted to a closed score which will be between 0 and 10. A minimum score of 5 is required to pass the written examination and proceed to the clinical examination (OSCE). The marking is computerized and feedback on performance is provided to those candidates who fail this part of the examination.

Objective Structured Clinical Examination (OSCE)

The OSCE was introduced for the first time in Spring 2003 and it replaced the individual patient assessment (i.e. the long case). The OSCE consists of 12 stations that test the range of psychiatric knowledge and skills acquired within first 12 months of basic specialist training (i.e. at the SHO level). The examination may include one or two additional pilot stations, the results of which do not count towards the overall result of the OSCE. The patient's role is played by a role player (actor/actress).

There is ONE examiner at each station, who observes the candidate as they perform their task. The examiner does not get involved except in exceptional circumstances. Candidates have ONE minute before entering each station to read the instructions. These include the purpose of the station and basic information about the patient, e.g. name, age, major symptoms. Each station has a number of predetermined objectives.

Time

Each station is of 7 minutes' duration and candidates must complete all stations. Thus the total duration of the OSCE circuit is 1 hour and 36 minutes, except when there are pilot or rest stations.

Marking system

The candidate is awarded a grade at each station. There are five grades from A to E:

A = excellent
B = good
C = average
D = fail
E = severe fail

Each objective (see above) is worth a percentage of the total marks for the station, which is calculated to give an overall grade for the station. Each candidate is required to demonstrate to the examiner that he or she has achieved a satisfactory standard of practice.

To pass the OSCE examination a minimum grade of C or above in at least nine of the 12 stations is generally required. A severe fail (grade E) in any station is considered as confirmation that the candidate did not attain the requisite standard in the OSCE.

2 OUTLINE OF THE WRITTEN PAPER

The ISQs were introduced in the MRCPsych I in Autumn 2001 and the EMIs were added in Spring 2003. The breakdown of ISQs in the papers in the book (as suggested by the Royal College of Psychiatrists) is a rough guide, intended to give candidates an idea of the areas of the curriculum that are covered by the examination. Questions on other areas of the curriculum may be included. The exact number of questions from each area is also a rough guide. There is no official breakdown that covers the EMI component of the paper.

Breakdown of ISQs

1 Basic sciences (39 questions)

Basic psychology	8
Behavioural psychology	10
Social psychology and neuropsychology	10
Human development	11

2 Psychopharmacology (23 questions)

General principles	5
Pharmacodynamics and pharmacokinetics	13
Adverse drug reactions	5

3 Psychopathology (45 questions)

Descriptive	39
Psychodynamic	6

4 Clinical theory and skills (26 questions)

Aetiology	6
Assessment and classification	6
History taking/interviewing	8
Mental state examination	4
Physical/neurological examination	2

3 OUTLINE OF THE CURRICULUM

The following outline is meant to be a quick checklist only. Candidates should refer to the Royal College of Psychiatrists Council Report CR95 (*CR95. Curriculum for basic specialist training and the MRCPsych examination*, 2001) for more information.

Basic sciences

Psychology

Basic psychology

- Principles of learning theory
- Auditory and visual perception
- Information processing and attention
- Memory, motivation, emotion
- Personality, thought processes
- Conscious, unconscious processes
- Intelligence
- Stress

Neuropsychology

- Organization of the brain in relation to memory, language, perception and visuospatial ability
- Functions of various parts of the brain
- Tests to measure various functions of the brain

Behavioural psychology

- Theory and applications of classical and operant conditioning
- Modelling, shaping
- Reinforcement, reciprocal inhibition
- Theory, principles and practice of cognitive–behavioural therapy

Social psychology

- Attitudes, interpersonal issues, intergroup behaviour
- Self-psychology, leadership, social influence, power and obedience
- Aggression, altruism and related matters

Psychological assessment

- Principles and methods of measurement

Human development

- Preconceptual and prenatal influences on development
- Life cycle theory, maturation, ageing

- Attachment and bonding, Bowlby's theory, types of attachment
- Influence of various adversities on child development
- Temperament, basic principles of emotional development
- Piaget's cognitive development theory, Erickson's theory, principles of language development, development of fears, anxiety, sexuality and gender role
- Principles of moral development: Freud's theory, Kohlberg's theory

Psychopharmacology

General principles of rational prescribing, classification, relation between the plasma drug level and therapeutic response.

Pharmacokinetics

- Principles of absorption, distribution, metabolism and elimination, with particular reference to oral, intramuscular and intravenous routes of administration
- Blood–brain barrier

Pharmacodynamics

- Main receptor subtypes, phenomena of receptor upregulation and downregulation
- Receptor signalling transduction mechanisms, e.g. G-proteins and the main messenger systems
- Adverse drug reactions
- Nature, prevalence/incidence of adverse drug reactions
- Drug interactions, common drug discontinuation reactions
- Controlled drugs

Psychopathology

Descriptive psychopathology

- Disorders of mood, thinking, perception, memory, self, consciousness, attention, concentration, body image
- Obsessive compulsive symptoms, depersonalization, derealization,
- Motor symptoms and signs
- Anxiety and phobic disorders, stress-related disorders
- Eating disorders, personality disorders, somatoform disorders
- Dissociative disorders

Dynamic psychopathology

- Defence mechanisms
- Theories of Freud, Jung, Klein, Winnicott, Adler
- Theories of neo-Freudians, e.g. Karen Horney, Erich Fromm, Harry Sullivan
- Interpretation of dreams

Clinical theory and skills

- Aetiology of mental disorders
- Classification of mental disorders
- History taking/interviewing
- Mental state examination
- Physical/neurological examination

4 ISQs AND EMIs AND HOW TO TACKLE THEM

Individual Statement Questions (ISQs)

These are single-stem statements with no relation to any of the other statements. However, there may be two or three consecutive statements on the same theme. Candidates are advised to consider each question on its own merit and answer as true or false. There is no negative marking in any part of the examination.

Preparing for ISQs

Candidates should review the core curriculum carefully and revise topics according to the number of questions per topic. For example, there are more questions from general adult psychiatry in the clinical topics paper; hence more attention should be paid to this topic. There is no substitute for extensive revision. A number of sources of ISQs and EMIs are available, including this book.

How to tackle ISQs

Candidates should give appropriate weight to each part of the paper according to the number of questions from each theme. Some candidates are good at psychology or dynamic psychopathology, whereas others might find them relatively more difficult. Hence, all candidates are advised to identify their weaknesses with practice papers and group revision well before the actual examination.

Extended Matching Items (EMIs)

Format

There are four elements in the structure of an EMI:

- Theme: This is a short title that focuses the candidate's attention on the subject of the question. For example, 'Management of depression'. It should help candidates to focus on a single, clear issue. The title will, therefore, encompass both the skills* and the knowledge** to be tested.
- Option list: This is a list of possible answers to the questions that follow; for example, the list may give a number of treatment options or diagnoses or clinical features. The list will be based on only one area of skill/knowledge and will NOT contain a mix of different areas, for example, diagnosis and treatment. The option list is therefore a homogeneous mix of items.
- Instructions (lead-in): This part tells the candidates about the task that has to be carried out.

- Questions: These are the problems which have to be solved by selecting the correct answers from the option list. Under each theme there are three questions.

*Skills: These include a variety of areas such as diagnostic skills, procedural skills, communication, bedside manners, etc.
**Knowledge: This covers the information acquired during the training period, for example, mood disorders, anxiety disorders, schizophrenia.

Reasons for the introduction of EMIs

The idea behind EMIs is to minimize the recognition effect that tends to occur in standard multiple choice question papers. This is achieved by the many possible combinations of vignettes and options. By using clinical cases instead of facts, the items can be used to test application of knowledge and problem-solving ability.

EMIs are easier to construct than key feature questions, as many questions can be drawn from one set of options, and the reliability has been shown to be good. EMIs are best when large numbers of similar kinds of decision, for example, relating to diagnosis or ordering of laboratory tests needs to be tested for different situations. EMIs are more likely to test clinical reasoning, that is, the application of clinical knowledge to practical situations.

The disadvantage of EMIs is that there is a risk of under-representation of certain themes simply because they do not fit the format of the test.

Skills and knowledge to be tested

- Diagnosis/differential diagnosis
- Clinical and procedural skills
- Investigations/selection and interpretation of diagnostic tests
- Management.

Context of clinical management

- Decisions supported by evidence including the principles of risk management, involving patients and, where appropriate, their relatives or carers in decisions about their care.
- Good practice in prescribing.
- Effective communicating skills including listening, questioning, explaining, involving patients in management, sharing information, recognizing that patients are knowledgeable, discussing options with patients and explaining the effects of treatment and procedures.
- Awareness and sensitivity of the need and expectations of patients regardless of their lifestyle, culture, beliefs, ethnicity, gender, sexuality, disability, age or social or economic status and understanding the patient's environment and its effects on their health.
- Disease factors such as inherited diseases and the natural history of disease.
- Practice of evidence-based medicine.
- Understanding of epidemiological principles and prevalence of important diseases in the UK.

- Awareness of methods of prevention and health promotion.
- Application of current scientific basis/understanding of mental disorders.
- Awareness of the different attitudes/behaviour that may be encountered in a multicultural society and appreciation of the impact of sociocultural factors on the incidence and prevalence of mental disorders.

Marking of EMIs

There are two types of EMI:

- R type, i.e. single best answer (3 marks)
- N type, i.e. multiple best answers
  - Two best answers (1.5 marks for each correct answer, total 3 marks)
  - Three best answers (1 mark for each correct answer, total 3 marks)

In questions with two and three best answers, only the first two and three answers, respectively, will be scored and the rest of the answers will be ignored.

How to tackle EMIs

Consider the range of topics under the heading 'Skills and knowledge to be tested'. Candidates should read the question first and then look for the answer(s) in the options list. Remember that the theme, i.e. the main area of the skills and knowledge being tested, informs what the EMI is about, e.g. diagnosis, investigations. This should help candidates to concentrate on the given exercise.

Remember that the questions require the best answer(s). Usually the number of correct answers for each question will be as required by the question. However, there may be other correct answers but which may not necessarily be the best answers. The majority of the EMIs will require the candidate to choose one best answer, and the rest will require two to three answers for each question.

5 EXPLANATION OF TERMS USED IN ISQ AND EMI PAPERS

Occurs	Does not give any indication of frequency of occurrence
Usually	60% or more
Recognized	Means it has been reported to occur as a feature or association
Characteristic	Features that occur often enough so as to be of some diagnostic value and whose absence might lead to doubts about the diagnosis
Diagnostic, essential and typical features	Must occur to make a diagnosis
Specific or pathognomonic	Features that occur in the named disease and no other
Can be or may be	Features are reported as occurring
Commonly, frequently, is likely or often	All imply a rate of occurrence greater than 50%
Particularly associated	Implies a significant association in some samples with sufficient numbers
Implicit	Implied although not plainly expressed
Explicit	Expressly stated
Exclusively	Features that occur in the named condition and no other
Invariably	Implies the occurrence of a feature without a shadow of doubt
Includes	Similar to 'occurs', i.e. makes no mention of frequency
Majority	More than 50%

6 OSCEs: AIMS, ADVANTAGES AND DISADVANTAGES

The OSCE is a series of highly structured and focused clinical assessment tasks through which candidates rotate in a systematic fashion. The aims of the OSCE are to test each candidate's clinical and communication skills, acquired within the first 12 months of basic specialist training. The present training requirement consists of 12 months in general adult psychiatry or 6 months in general adult psychiatry and 6 months in old age psychiatry. The examiner observes the candidate putting his or her skills into practice.

OSCEs reduce the 'luck of the draw' in selection of examiners and patients in the outcome of postgraduate examination in psychiatry, particularly for those candidates who are on the pass/fail borderline. The OSCE allows the Royal College of Psychiatrists to assess the areas of clinical practice which could not be examined in the traditional long case. For example, ability to communicate diagnosis, investigations, treatment and prognosis to patients and their carers; physical examination; interpretation of results; communicating complex clinical judgements to other clinicians, including nurses, physicians, surgeons and other colleagues.

Historical perspective

The objective structured clinical examination was first described by Harden and Gleeson (1970) as 'a timed examination in which medical students interact with a series of simulated patients in stations that may involve history taking, physical examination, counselling or patient management'. Simulated or standardized patients have been used in medical examinations and other medical settings for more than 30 years, including in undergraduate and postgraduate training (communication and clinical skills), monitoring of doctors' performance and standardization of clinical examination. Simulation has been used in the industry and military for much longer (Jason et al., 1971).

The Royal College of Psychiatrists introduced OSCEs to replace the individual patient assessment ('long case') in the clinical component of the MRCPsych Part I examination with a view to increasing the reliability and validity of the clinical examination (see www.rcpsych.ac.uk/traindev/exams/regulation/summarycurrent.htm) in Spring 2003.

Although the terms 'simulated' or 'standardized' have different meanings, they are often used interchangeably. 'Standardized' patients are real or simulated patients who have been coached to present a clinical problem (Vu and Barrow, 1994). 'Simulated' patients are not a homogeneous group as they can come from a variety of backgrounds. Their only common characteristic is that of simulating real patients. In the MRCPsych examination, the simulated patients are professionally trained actors/actresses playing the role of patients.

Advantages of OSCEs

- Simulation of real-life situations.
- They can simultaneously engage the qualities of reality and be explicitly controlled and safe.
- Simulated patients can give direct feedback to the candidates on their performance.
- Patients are readily available when required.
- They allow different candidates to be presented with a similar challenge, thereby reducing an important source of variability (Norman *et al.*, 1985).
- Stations can be tailored to the level of skills to be assessed.
- Scenarios that are distressing to real patients can be simulated.
- The patient variable in the examination is uniform across candidates.
- They allow wide areas of skills to be tested and reduce the impact of any one examiner on the overall outcome of one candidate.
- More valid examinations than the traditional approach to clinical examination.
- The examiners can decide in advance what is to be tested and then can design examinations to test those competencies.
- The content and complexities can be adjusted according to the stages of training of the candidates.
- A large sample of candidates' skills and a large number of candidates can be tested.

Disadvantages of OSCEs

- The idealized 'textbook' scenarios may not mimic real life.
- They may not allow assessment of complex clinical skills.
- Resource intensive.
- Time consuming.
- Training issues in setting up stations.
- Demanding for both the examiners and simulated patients who are required to pay close attention to candidates repeating the same tasks on a number of occasions.

Possible problems with OSCEs in psychiatry

It has been comparatively more difficult to achieve reliability and validity of OSCEs in psychiatry examinations for the following reasons:

- The binary checklists typically used in most OSCEs are insufficiently sensitive to detect higher clinical components, such as empathy, rapport and ethics (Cox, 1990).
- Although a typical OSCE station lasts up to 7 minutes, a traditional psychiatric interview takes 50 minutes, raising questions about the content validity of the short OSCE station.
- Complex psychiatric presentations, such as thought disorder, are difficult to simulate (Hodges *et al.*, 1998).
- This runs the risk of training doctors who are very good at performing these piecemeal tasks without being able to assimilate them into a coherent assessment.
- It could be argued that the skills required to deal with a single case and make sense of it in all its complexities are not examined.

7 SKILLS TO BE TESTED IN OSCEs

- Communication skills: There will be a communication element in most stations. However, in some stations, this will be the principal skill tested.
- History taking.
- Clinical examination skills: The candidates are asked to examine a particular part of the body of simulated patients or perform the examination on an anatomical model. They should ONLY take a history or perform the examination according to instructions. They may be asked to explain their actions to the patients and/or examiners.
- Practical skills/use of equipment: This is to assess some of the practical skills a senior house officer or equivalent trainee needs to possess. The stations concerned will normally involve anatomical models rather than patients.
- Emergency management: These stations will test whether the candidates know what to do in an emergency situation. The candidates may be asked to explain what they are doing either to the patient or to the examiner.

8 FORMAT OF OSCEs

There are 12 booths known as 'stations'. Each station requires candidates to undertake a particular task. Some tasks involve talking to or examining patients, some involve demonstrating a procedure on an anatomical model, whereas others involve watching a video clip and recognizing clinical phenomena.

There may be up to two rest stations in the circuit. There may also be pilot stations containing instructions asking the candidates to perform certain tasks as if they were at a real station. The results of these stations do not count towards a candidate's overall OSCE grades.

All candidates are required to go to all 12 stations and perform all tasks. Each task lasts 7 minutes. A bell rings after 6 minutes to warn candidates of the time left and another bell rings when the 7 minutes are up. Each station has one examiner. In general, candidates are not required to have a conversation with the examiner. They should only direct their remarks to the examiner if the instructions specifically ask them to do so. If a candidate finishes the task before the 7 minutes are up, they must wait inside the station. They should not speak to the examiner or to the patient during this time.

Candidate instructions are posted outside each station and they are also available in each station. Candidates wait outside the next station for 1 minute. During this time they should read the instructions for the task to be undertaken in that station.

9 MARKING OF OSCEs

OSCEs are particularly suited to criterion-referenced examinations, where a pass/fail decision has to be taken, and where a decision has to be made as to whether a student has reached a prescribed standard and is able to graduate or pass on to the next part of training/course.

The marking schedule is not binary in nature. It is a 5-point scale that is also used in other medical Royal College examinations in the UK. OSCEs are objectively marked, i.e. there is weighting of particular objectives in each OSCE station that is predetermined and the examiner's task is to award a mark for each objective as mentioned on the mark sheet. The examiners are not aware of the weighting for each task.

The candidates pass or fail mark is determined by his or her performance on these objectives and their relative weightings. Marking does not include the opinions of simulated patients. All OSCE stations usually have communication skills as one of the objectives.

10 PREPARING FOR OSCEs

Candidates should start thinking about OSCEs in the first six months of their basic specialist training. The following lists should be useful for candidates when preparing for OSCEs with the help of their colleagues. The lists are not exhaustive but cover the commonly asked questions and exercises.

Communication skills

- Active listening.
- Involving patients/carers in decision making and checking their understanding.
- Communicating with other healthcare professionals, e.g. discussing a patient with a senior medical colleague.
- Breaking bad news, building rapport and showing empathy, respect and sensitivity to others' emotions and coping with strong emotions of other people.
- Seeking informed consent for investigations, electroconvulsive therapy (ECT), antimanic drugs, antipsychotic depot injections, clozapine.
- Dealing with anxious or angry patients or carers.
- Giving instructions on discharge from hospital.
- Giving advice on lifestyle, health promotion or risk factors.
- Dealing with complaints.
- Explaining cognitive–behavioural therapy and other psychological treatments for depression, anxiety disorders, psychotic symptoms, eating disorders.
- Explaining counselling, psychodynamic therapy, cognitive analytic therapy, interpersonal therapy, family therapy, group therapy.
- Explaining diagnosis and prognosis of common mental disorders, e.g. schizophrenia, depression, bipolar affective disorder, dementia, eating disorders, anxiety disorders, substance misuse and dependence.
- Explaining investigations, e.g. tests for clozapine and lithium therapy, preparation for ECT, brain imaging, etc.
- Explaining treatment (acute, maintenance, i.e. to prevent relapse, and prophylaxis, i.e. to prevent recurrence):
  - Antidepressant drugs
  - Antipsychotic drugs including depot injections and clozapine
  - Antimanic (mood stabilizer) drugs
  - Antidementia drugs in mild, moderate and severe dementias
  - Drug treatment in special situations, e.g. antidepressants, antipsychotic and antimanic drugs in pregnancy and puerperium.
- Explaining detention and treatment under the Mental Health Act 1983.
- Assessing a mute patient.
- Assessing the capacity to consent to psychiatric treatment and surgical/medical procedures or treatments.

- Liaising with general hospital colleagues regarding disturbed patients.
- Explaining driving regulations in relation to recent episodes of severe depression and psychosis, drug and alcohol dependence, etc.
- Explaining drug treatment in pregnancy, puerperium, children and elderly persons.

History taking

- Eliciting psychotic symptoms, including Schneider's first rank symptoms from patients with schizophrenia, schizoaffective disorder, mania, depression, persistent delusional disorder, etc.
- Eliciting delusional beliefs.
- Eliciting hallucinatory experiences.
- Eliciting salient features of mood disorders, e.g. depression, mania.
- Eliciting negative cognitions in depression.
- Eliciting features of normal, abnormal and prolonged grief reactions.
- Eliciting salient features of anxiety disorders, e.g. panic disorder, agoraphobia, social phobia, specific phobias, obsessive compulsive disorder, generalized anxiety disorder.
- Eliciting salient features of post-traumatic stress disorder, adjustment disorders and stress reactions.
- Eliciting features of anorexia and bulimia nervosa with or without co-morbidity, such as type I diabetes mellitus (insulin-dependent diabetes mellitus).
- Eliciting salient features of alcohol and drug misuse as well as dependence.
- Eliciting features of frontotemporal dementia, Alzheimer's disease, multi-infarct dementia, Lewy body dementia, Pick's disease, Creutzfeldt–Jakob disease, Huntington's disease, Parkinson's disease and multiple disseminated sclerosis.
- Eliciting salient features of schizoid, schizotypal, antisocial (dissocial), and borderline (emotionally unstable), histrionic and narcissistic personality disorders.
- Eliciting salient features of somatoform disorders, e.g. somatization, hypochondria, persistent somatoform pain disorder.
- Eliciting features of body dysmorphic disorder, transsexualism, dual-role transvestism, fetishism, fetishistic transvestism, exhibitionism, premature ejaculation, erectile impotence, etc.
- Eliciting history of sexual dysfunction of a patient on psychotropic drugs from his or her partner.
- Assessing risk of deliberate self-harm and suicide in a variety of settings, e.g. accident and emergency, general hospital wards, police station.
- Assessing risk of aggression/violence in a variety of settings, e.g. accident and emergency, out-patient clinic, reception area, general hospital wards, police station.

- Assessing risk in patients with memory disorders.
- Eliciting features of chronic fatigue syndrome, morbid jealousy, sleep disorders, depersonalization.
- Eliciting symptoms of post-natal depression, maternity blues, puerperal psychosis.
- Risk assessment in the above patients.
- Eliciting collateral history from relatives/carers regarding schizophrenia, depression, bipolar affective disorder, dementia, substance misuse, etc.
- Eliciting history of seizures in a patient on clozapine, phenothiazines or tricyclic and other antidepressant drugs.
- Assessing compliance of patients suffering from long-term mental illnesses.
- Assessing a patient's wellbeing in the clinical setting.

Clinical examination skills

The candidates are assessed on their ability to conduct a physical examination of simulated patients. In certain circumstances, the examination will be carried out on a manikin or model. They should only take a history or make a diagnosis if instructions require them to do so. They may be asked to explain their actions to the examiner and the patient as they go along. Examples include:

- Cranial nerves
- Motor and sensory nervous systems
- Extrapyramidal side effects
- Fundi
- Signs of alcohol and drug dependence
- Mini-Mental State Examination
- Assessing cognitive functions in elderly persons, Wernicke–Korsakoff syndrome
- Assessing nature, form and content of thought disorders
- Assessing frontal lobe functions
- Assessing dominant and non-dominant hemisphere functions
- Performing cardiovascular examination, especially risk factors for vascular dementia
- Examining patients with possible eating disorders and thyroid dysfunction

Practical skills and use of equipment

These stations assess some of the practical skills an SHO would have learnt during the first year of training. The stations concerned will usually involve anatomical models rather than patients. The candidates must also be able to use appropriate equipment when carrying out an examination.

- Determination of correct settings on an ECT apparatus
- Application of ECT electrodes

- Application of ECG leads
- Interpreting ECG, electroencephalogram (EEG), blood tests, radiographs, computed tomography (CT) and magnetic resonance imaging (MRI) scans

Emergency management

- Cardiopulmonary resuscitation (CPR)
- Control and restraint
- Rapid tranquillization.

11 HOW TO TACKLE OSCEs

Some guidelines for a successful performance in the domains discussed in the previous section are given below.

Communication skills

Candidates should keep the following examples in mind when undertaking the OSCE for communication skills.

Explaining schizophrenia to a relative

Construct: This station tests the candidate's ability to establish rapport with a distressed relative.

Main issues to be covered:

- Explaining the aetiology, nature, signs and symptoms and prognosis of schizophrenia.
- Explaining pharmacological and psychosocial treatments.
- Explaining risks associated with the illness.
- Establishing the relative's beliefs, concerns, fears and expectations and addressing them.
- Explaining in a way that the relative understands, giving balanced, accurate and realistic information with instillation of hope.

Consent to ECT

Construct: This station tests the candidate's ability to give sufficient information to the patient to assist him or her to arrive at a decision whether to accept ECT or not.

Main issues to be covered:

- Explaining the nature and purpose of ECT.
- Explaining the procedure of ECT including blood tests, electrocardiogram (ECG), etc.
- Explaining how it works.
- Explaining potential benefits, adverse effects and alternatives to ECT.
- Explaining whether the Mental Health Act can be invoked or not.
- Establishing patient's beliefs, concerns, fears and expectations and addressing them.

History taking

Candidates should keep the following examples in mind in answering OSCEs for history taking.

Assessing a patient in the context of the Mental Health Act

Construct: This station tests the ability to assess a patient's admission to hospital under the Mental Health Act or not.

Main issues to be covered:

- Whether the patient is mentally disordered (mental illness, mental impairment, severe mental impairment or psychopathic disorder) or not.
- The nature and/or degree of the mental disorder.
- The risk factors such as risk to patient's own health, own safety and/or protection of other persons, whether the patient is able to safeguard against exploitation and self-neglect.
- Whether the proposed treatment is likely to alleviate patient's suffering or prevent deterioration of health.
- Alternatives to hospitalization in a less restrictive environment.
- Insight into mental health problems and willingness to cooperate with the professionals.

History of bulimia nervosa

Construct: This station tests the candidate's ability to elicit clinical features of bulimia nervosa.

Main issues to be covered:

- Presenting complaints
- Characteristic features of bulimia
- Differentiation of bulimia from anorexia nervosa
- Explaining diagnosis to the patient.

History taking in postnatal depression

Construct: This station assesses the candidate's ability to take a history that will establish the diagnosis of postnatal depression.

Main issues to be covered:

- History of salient features of depression
- Differentiation from maternity blues, and puerperal psychosis
- Assessment of risk to self and the infant
- Past psychiatric history if applicable.

Clinical examination

Candidates should keep the following examples in mind in OSCEs about clinical examination.

Assessing frontal lobe functions

Construct: This station assesses the candidate's ability to test frontal lobe functions by performing simple bedside tests.

- The candidate should look for over-familiarity, disinhibition, irritability, distractibility, apathy, lack of emotional concern and perseveration.
- Test for motor control and the ability to initiate a task and to follow a sequence of instructions, for example, finger–nose–finger task, Go/No go tasks, Luria hand sequence.
- Test for abstract reasoning (e.g. a proverb test), fluency (e.g. naming words beginning with letter A, B, C, etc.), and cognitive estimates (e.g. What is the best paid job in the UK? What is the average height of British women?).
- Test for primitive reflexes.

Assessing capacity to consent

Construct: This station tests the candidate's ability to assess the patient's capacity to consent and liaise with other professionals.

Main issues to be covered include the ability to assess the patient's:

- understanding of the problem/matter in hand
- understanding of the nature and purpose of the proposed procedure or treatment
- understanding the benefits/risks of the proposed procedure or treatment
- understanding of the risks of not having the proposed procedure or treatment
- ability to believe in the given information
- ability to consider pros and cons of the information so as to arrive at a decision.

References

Cox K (1990) No Oscar for OSCE. *Med Educ* 24, 540–545.
Harden RM, Gleeson FA (1970) Assessment of clinical competence using objective structured clinical examination (OSCE). *Med Educ* 13, 41–54.
Hodges B, Regehr G, Hanson M *et al.* (1998) Validation of objective structured clinical examination in psychiatry. *Acad Med* 73, 910–912.
Jason H, Kagan N, Werner A *et al.* (1971) New approaches to teaching basic interview skills to medical students. *Am J Psychiatry* 127, 140–142.

Norman GR, Burrows HS, Gliva G *et al.* (1985) Simulated patients. In: VR Neufield, GR Norman (eds). *Assessing Clinical Competence.* New York: Springer.

Vu NV, Barrow HS (1994) Use of standardized patients in clinical assessments: recent developments and measurement findings. *Educ Res* **23**, 23–30.

SECTION 2:
PAPERS

PAPER 1 ISQs

Questions

Basic sciences

Basic psychology

1   Schedules of reinforcement include fixed interval schedules.

2   Schedules of reinforcement include fixed reinforcement schedules.

3   Schedules of reinforcement include variable reinforcement schedules.

4   Schedules of reinforcement include fixed ratio schedules.

5   Schedules of reinforcement include variable ratio schedules.

6   In cognitive theory, the term 'cognition' is used in reference to cognitive events.

7   In cognitive theory, the term 'cognition' is used in reference to cognitive attitudes.

8   In cognitive theory, the term 'cognition' is used in reference to cognitive beliefs.

9   In cognitive theory, the term 'cognition' is used in reference to cognitive processes.

10 In cognitive theory, the term 'cognition' is used in reference to cognitive structures.

11 The cognitive–behavioural model of depression gives primacy to emotional states that give rise to cognitions.

12 In self-serving attributional bias, one's own failures are attributed to situational factors.

13 Backward conditioning is a type of classical conditioning.

14 Maslow's hierarchy of needs includes spiritual reflection.

15 The Bender Gestalt Test is a test of visuo-motor coordination.

16 According to the attribution theory, people tend to attribute their behaviour to their personality traits.

17 According to learning theory, covert desensitization is a method of increasing the frequency of a behaviour by associating it with imagery of unpleasant consequences.

18   According to learning theory, classical conditioning occurs rapidly upon repeated priming of stimuli.

19   Nomothetic approaches consider behaviour of individual persons as unique to them.

20   A personality trait is defined as an enduring characteristic feature of an individual.

21   Visual imagery during encoding improves retrieval of memorized information.

22   Retrieval of information presented early in a word list is called the 'primacy' effect.

23   According to the modal model of memory, information passes from short-term memory to long-term memory.

24   Procedural memory is explicit in nature.

25   Bottom-up processing results in constructive memories.

26   According to the Cannon–Bard theory, felt emotions depend upon interpretation of the general state of bodily arousal.

27   Imprinting is unaffected by environmental factors.

28   Learned helplessness is an example of classical conditioning.

29   Habituation is a form of adaptation.

30   Habituation is an all or none phenomenon.

31   Cognitive dissonance can arise from logical reasons.

32   Cognitive dissonance is considered affectively neutral.

33   Cognitive dissonance can be reduced by dismissing or denying information.

[answers on page 43]

Behavioural psychology

34   The cognitive–behavioural model of depression was influenced by the work of Albert Ellis.

35   The cognitive–behavioural model of depression uses the concept of schema.

36   The cognitive–behavioural model of depression includes Beck's depressive triad.

37   The cognitive–behavioural model of depression suggests that events play no part in the occurrence of depression.

38   The cognitive triad of depression includes a negative expectation of the future.

39   In learning theory, Premack's principle states that behaviour engaged at a higher frequency can be used to reinforce low-frequency behaviour.

40   Negative reinforcement is a process by which a response that leads to removal of an aversive event is decreased.

41   Punishment is an aversive stimulus that is presented specifically to weaken an undesirable response.

[answers on page 44]

Neuropsychology

42   The Halstead Category Test is used to detect disturbances of reasoning, abstraction and logical analysis.

43   According to learning theory, anxiety is a conditioned response to specific environmental stimuli.

44   Broca's aphasia is associated with lesions of the third frontal gyrus of the non-dominant hemisphere.

45   The Halstead–Reitan battery test has a sensitivity in the order of 99 per cent to presence of brain damage.

46   The Luria–Nebraska battery test has a sensitivity in the order of 95 per cent to the presence of brain damage.

47   In Broca's aphasia, speech is characteristically slowed, hesitant, laborious and particularly marked by agrammatism.

48   In Wernicke's aphasia, speech is characteristically rapid and fluent with largely preserved syntax.

49   In jargon aphasia, speech is replete with word substitutions and neologisms.

50   The term 'prosopagnosia' refers to the inability to recognize familiar faces.

51   In psychogenic amnesia, the sense of personal identity and autobiographical memory are preserved.

[answers on page 44]

Human development

52   Jean Piaget is best known for his theories on the development of intelligence.

53   Jean Piaget is best known for his theories on the roots of human aggression.

54   The nature of the relationship between a child and their caregiver is not affected by the state and temperament of both.

55   A developmentally delayed or irritable child will not respond to the overtures of the caregiver.

56   Formation of an attachment between an infant and the caregiver seems to rely on instant recognition or attraction.

57   The attachment relationship is based on reciprocal interaction rather than upon the meeting or satisfaction of physical needs.

58   According to Bowlby, although there is generally a primary attachment, a hierarchy of attachment figures is formed.

59   According to Piaget's theory of cognitive development, lack of object permanence is a characteristic feature of the sensorimotor stage.

60   According to Piaget's theory of cognitive development, primary circular reactions are seen during the preoperational stage.

61   According to Piaget's theory of cognitive development, secondary circular reactions occur during the sensorimotor stage.

62   According to Piaget's theory of cognitive development, tertiary circular reactions occur during the operational stage.

63   According to Piaget's theory of cognitive development, concrete operational children are egocentric.

[answers on page 44]

Psychopharmacology

General principles

64   Risperidone is a benzisoxazole derivative.

65   Risperidone acts as an antagonist at D2 receptors.

66   Risperidone acts as an agonist at S2 receptors.

67   Risperidone has no clinically significant actions on noradrenergic and histaminergic receptors.

[answers on page 45]

Pharmacokinetics

68   With regard to the pharmacokinetic properties of diazepam, its elimination half-life is 10 times greater in elderly people than in young adults.

69   With regard to the pharmacokinetic properties of benzodiazepines, there is only 50 per cent availability after oral administration.

70   With regard to the pharmacokinetic properties of benzodiazepines, there is 50 per cent protein binding.

71   With regard to the pharmacokinetic properties of diazepam, desmethyldiazepam is an inactive metabolite.

72   With regard to the pharmacokinetic properties of diazepam, the presence of food reduces the extent of absorption.

73   With regard to the physiological effects of benzodiazepines at therapeutic doses, they have little effect on autonomic functions.

74   With regard to the physiological effects of benzodiazepines, they induce hepatic microsomal enzymes.

75   With reference to the physiological effects of benzodiazepines, the dexamethasone suppression test is usually unaffected.

76   With reference to the physiological effects of benzodiazepines, inhibition of the afferent pathways in the spinal cord results in skeletal muscle relaxation.

77   With reference to physiological effects of benzodiazepines, neuroendocrine systems are not affected.

[answers on page 45]

Pharmacodynamics

78   With reference to excitatory amino acid receptors, *N*-methyl-D-aspartate (NMDA) receptor activity is modulated by chloride ions.

79   With reference to excitatory amino acid receptors, phencyclidine acts as an agonist at the NMDA-linked ion channel.

80   With reference to excitatory amino acid receptors, NMDA receptors are found in high concentrations in the raphe nuclei.

81   With reference to excitatory amino acid receptors, epileptic fits may occur as a result of sudden release of glycine.

82   With reference to excitatory amino acid receptors, neuronal death due to the toxic effects of glutamate has been implicated in cerebral ischaemia.

[answers on page 45]

Adverse drug reactions

83   Risperidone has an increased liability to produce extrapyramidal symptoms compared with haloperidol.

84   The patient who is breast-feeding should avoid amitriptyline.

85   The patient who is breast-feeding should avoid sulpiride.

86   The patient who is breast-feeding should avoid carbamazepine.

87   The patient who is breast-feeding should avoid lithium carbonate.

88   The patient who is breast-feeding should avoid sertraline.

89   Long-term treatment with fluoxetine causes significant weight gain in a majority of patients.

90   Long-term treatment with carbamazepine causes significant weight gain in a majority of patients.

91   Long-term treatment with moclobemide causes significant weight gain in a majority of patients.

92   Long-term treatment with diazepam causes significant weight gain in a majority of patients.

93   Long-term treatment with risperidone causes significant weight gain in a majority of patients.

94   Visual accommodation may be adversely affected by chlordiazepoxide in therapeutic doses.

95   Visual accommodation may be adversely affected by dothiepin in therapeutic doses.

96   Visual accommodation may be adversely affected by sertraline in therapeutic doses.

97   Visual accommodation may be adversely affected by trazodone in therapeutic doses.

98   Visual accommodation may be adversely affected by benztropine in therapeutic doses.

[answers on page 46]

Psychopathology

Descriptive

99   Catatonia occurs exclusively in patients with schizophrenia.

100   Catatonia is a common presentation in conversion disorders.

101   Catatonia includes the phenomenon of 'Mitmachen'.

102   Catatonia includes the phenomenon of 'Gedankenlautwerden'.

103   Catatonia was first described by Kasanin.

104   Parsimony is a characteristic feature of obsessional personality.

105   Lack of adaptability to new situations is a characteristic feature of obsessional personality.

106   Obstinacy is a characteristic feature of obsessional personality.

107   Persistent difficulty in establishing a sexual relationship is a characteristic feature of obsessional personality.

108 Indecisiveness is a characteristic feature of obsessional personality.

109 A typical features of the pathological grief reaction is the bereaved person searching for the deceased person.

110 A typical feature of the pathological grief reaction is visual hallucinations.

111 A typical feature of the pathological grief reaction is denial.

112 A typical feature of the pathological grief reaction is auditory hallucinations.

113 A typical feature of the pathological grief reaction is resurrection of the deceased person's last illness.

114 In the hysterical conversion syndrome, the symptoms usually reduce conscious anxiety.

115 In the hysterical conversion syndrome, a history of histrionic personality is found in almost all patients.

116 In the hysterical conversion syndrome, symptoms are mediated via the autonomic nervous system.

117 In the hysterical conversion syndrome, symptoms disappear as soon as the primary gain is achieved.

118 In the hysterical conversion syndrome, the symptoms are symbolic representations of intrapsychic conflicts.

119 Typical features of malingering include the ultimate resolution of symptoms when the claim is settled.

120 Typical features of malingering include frontal headaches.

121 Typical features of malingering include fainting attacks.

122 Typical features of malingering include severe difficulties with sleep.

123 Typical features of malingering include seeking financial compensation after sustaining a relatively major injury.

124 All delusions are essentially delusions of reference in that they relate to the patient and/or others.

125 Delusions are always associated with loss of ego boundaries.

126 A delusion is an invariably false belief held against the evidence to the contrary.

127 Delusional perception is pathognomonic of schizophrenia in the absence of organic brain disease.

128 Presence of olfactory hallucinations is compatible with the diagnosis of persistent delusional disorder.

129 Auditory hallucinations in clear consciousness occur in atropine poisoning.

130 Presence of persistent auditory hallucinations is compatible with the diagnosis of persistent delusional disorders.

131 Presence of tactile hallucinations is compatible with the diagnosis of persistent delusional disorders.

132 Auditory hallucinations in clear consciousness occur in cocaine abuse.

133 Auditory hallucinations in clear consciousness occur in mushroom poisoning.

134 Eidetic images are essentially visual hallucinations.

135 Eidetic images are never perceived in relation to a real object.

136 Eidetic images may be thought of as 'photographic memory'.

137 Eidetic images are a form of extracampine visual hallucinations.

138 Eidetic images can be called up and terminated by voluntary effort.

139 In the first month of bereavement, morbid rather than normal grief is indicated by persistent denial of loss.

140 In the first month of bereavement, morbid rather than normal grief is indicated by recurrent panic attacks.

141 In the first month of bereavement, morbid rather than normal grief is indicated by self-blame.

142 In the first month of bereavement, morbid rather than normal grief is indicated by recurrent nightmares involving the deceased.

143 In the first month of bereavement, morbid rather than normal grief is indicated by searching behaviour.

144 Factors that significantly increase the risk of suicide in a patient with schizophrenia include thought echo.

145 Presence of akathisia significantly increases the risk of suicide in a patient with schizophrenia.

146 Factors which significantly increase the risk of suicide in a patient with schizophrenia include fear of mental disorientation.

147 Factors which significantly increase the risk of suicide in a patient with schizophrenia include unemployment.

148 High premorbid educational attainment significantly increases the risk of suicide in a patient with schizophrenia.

149 Overeating is a recognized feature of anorexia nervosa.

150 Overeating is a recognized feature of agoraphobia.

151 Overeating is a recognized feature of social phobia.

152 Overeating is a recognized feature of bulimia nervosa.

153 Overeating is a recognized feature of depression.

154 Clinical features of normal-weight bulimia include abdominal striae.

155 Clinical features of normal-weight bulimia include lanugo hair.

156 Clinical features of normal-weight bulimia include bradycardia.

157 Clinical features of normal-weight bulimia include erosion of tooth enamel.

158 Clinical features of normal-weight bulimia include calluses on the fingers.

159 Night terrors occur in stage IV of orthodox sleep.

160 Night terrors are genetically linked to sleepwalking.

161 Night terrors occur in the first half of sleep during the night.

162 Night terrors are associated with slow alpha rhythm in electroencephalograph (EEG) recordings.

163 Night terrors occur exclusively in rapid eye movement (REM) sleep.

164 Autochthonous delusions are usually persecutory in nature.

165 The paranoid-schizoid position in an infant implies developmental delay.

166 The paranoid-schizoid position in an infant implies ambivalence towards the mother.

167 An overvalued idea is an unpleasant and sustained false belief which dominates a person's life.

168 Thought broadcasting means that thoughts are being removed from a person's mind by other people.

169 The terms 'micropsia' and 'Lilliputian hallucinations' are interchangeable.

[answers on page 46]

Psychodynamic

170 In dynamic psychopathology, 'paranosic' gain is environmental and can be shaped by culture and society.

171 In dynamic psychopathology, 'paranosic' gain is the immediate consequence of defence processes.

172 In dynamic psychopathology, 'paranosic' gain is a means of discharging tension created by intrapsychic conflicts.

173 In dynamic psychopathology, 'paranosic' gain is a temporary freedom from work demands.

174 In dynamic psychopathology, 'paranosic' gain results in impulse control.

175 Transference is the experience of a feeling towards a person that does not befit the person but belongs to another person in the past.

176 Transference is interpreted thoroughly in supportive psychotherapy.

177 Transference is a response to the therapist's countertransference.

178 Transference can be differentiated from countertransference by its degree and character.

179 Transference is thoroughly analysed in psychoanalytic psychotherapy.

180 The recognized ego defence mechanisms in obsessive–compulsive disorder include denial.

181 The recognized ego defence mechanisms in obsessive–compulsive disorder include magic doing and undoing.

182 The recognized ego defence mechanisms in obsessive–compulsive disorder include suppression.

183 The recognized ego defence mechanisms in obsessive–compulsive disorder include reaction formation.

184 The recognized ego defence mechanisms in obsessive–compulsive disorder include isolation.

185 According to Freud's model of the mind, the id is the most destructive element of the mind.

186 According to Freud's model of the mind, the ego functions by a conscious process.

187 According to Freud's model of the mind, the id is the primary source of libidinal energy.

188 According to Freud's model of the mind, the superego functions by means of secondary process thinking.

189 According to Freud's model of the mind, the id functions entirely by an unconscious process.

190 As regards dynamic psychotherapy, it aims to offer an opportunity for a transference relationship to grow and develop.

191 Dynamic psychotherapy inevitably contains a behavioural modification component.

192 Dynamic psychotherapy is mainly concerned with neurotic symptoms.

193 Dynamic psychotherapy aims to offer an opportunity for counter transference to grow and develop.

194 Dynamic psychotherapy involves exclusive analysis of the patient's characteristic defence mechanisms.

195 According to Freud's psychoanalytic theory, the id functions by means of primary process thinking.

196 According to Freud's psychoanalytic theory, the id functions by means of tertiary process thinking.

197 According to Freud's psychoanalytic theory, the id aims at immediate release of tension without regard for the consequences.

198 According to Freud's psychoanalytic theory, the superego is the conscience of the individual.

199 According to Freud's psychoanalytic theory, the id obeys reality principles.

200 As regards brief dynamic psychotherapy, focalization of the conflict is an essential feature.

201 As regards brief dynamic psychotherapy, the termination date is set in advance in all types of such therapies.

202 As regards brief dynamic psychotherapy, it is most helpful in circumscribed neurotic problems.

203 As regards brief dynamic psychotherapy, Malan and Horowitz are the leading proponents.

204 As regards brief dynamic psychotherapy, its indications include patients with interpersonal relationship difficulties.

[answers on page 48]

Clinical theory and skills

Aetiology

205 Central retinal vein thrombosis is a recognized cause of papilloedema.

206 Hypoparathyroidism is a recognized cause of papilloedema.

207 Cavernous sinus thrombosis is a recognized cause of papilloedema.

208 Hypercapnia is a recognized cause of papilloedema.

209 Temporal arteritis is a recognized cause of papilloedema.

210 Short-lived paranoid psychosis with auditory hallucinations is likely to be caused by the use of barbiturates.

211   Short-lived paranoid psychosis with auditory hallucinations is likely to be caused by the use of procyclidine.

212   Short-lived paranoid psychosis with auditory hallucinations is likely to be caused by the use of cannabis.

213   Short-lived paranoid psychosis with auditory hallucinations is likely to be caused by the use of alcohol.

214   Short-lived paranoid psychosis with auditory hallucinations is likely to be caused by use of lysergic acid diethylamide (LSD).

[answers on page 50]

Classification/diagnosis

215   Classification of mental disorders based on aetiology includes delirium tremens.

216   Classification of mental disorders based on aetiology includes Wilson's disease.

217   Classification of mental disorders based on aetiology includes Korsakoff's disease.

218   Classification of mental disorders based on aetiology includes Alzheimer's disease.

219   Classification of mental disorders based on aetiology includes Briquet's syndrome.

220   As regards the classification of mental disorders, most of them have pathognomonic symptoms.

221   As regards the classification of mental disorders, the symptoms used to define a disorder can be reliably elicited.

222   As regards the classification of mental disorders, the diagnosis is usually based on a group of symptoms.

223   As regards the classification of mental disorders, external validity of most psychiatric diagnoses is high.

224   As regards the classification of mental disorders, one based on psychodynamic principles would be the most reliable.

225   As regards the International Classification of Diseases (ICD-10), it categorizes alcohol abuse separately from abuse of other drugs.

226   As regards ICD-10, the number of categories containing the diagnosis of depression has been nearly halved in comparison with ICD-9.

227   As regards ICD-10, it continues to distinguish between psychoses and neuroses.

228 As regards ICD-10, the final draft was produced after field trials.

229 As regards ICD-10, the field trials were much more extensive than those used for ICD-9.

[answers on page 50]

History taking/interviewing

230 Objective evidence of a patient's feelings during an interview can be divulged by observing his or her facial expression.

231 Objective evidence of a patient's feelings during an interview can be divulged by his or her motor behaviour.

232 Objective evidence of a patient's feelings during an interview can be divulged by the patient's stated feelings.

233 Objective evidence of a patient's feelings during an interview can be divulged by the pattern of speech.

234 Objective evidence of a patient's feelings during an interview can be divulged by his or her emotional behaviour during the interview.

235 As regards techniques used during a psychiatric interview, reflection refers to the exact repetition of what the patient has said.

236 As regards techniques used during a psychiatric interview, direct questions seek information of a non-specific nature.

237 As regards techniques used during a psychiatric interview, confrontation refers to a technique in which further information and explanation are elicited from a patient.

238 As regards techniques used during a psychiatric interview, silence should be avoided at all possible costs.

239 As regards techniques used during a psychiatric interview, recapitulation should be used at the beginning of the interview.

240 The interviewer's behaviour during an interview, which could lead to an inadequate disclosure by the patient, includes normalization.

241 The interviewer's behaviour during an interview, which could lead to an inadequate disclosure by the patient, includes premature reassurance.

242 The interviewer's behaviour during an interview, which could lead to an inadequate disclosure by the patient, includes open-ended questions.

243 The interviewer's behaviour during an interview, which could lead to an inadequate disclosure by the patient, includes false reassurance.

244 The assessment of patients with schizophrenia must take into account third party information as far as possible.

245   Up to 45 per cent of patients suffering from bipolar affective disorder
       have a history of substance misuse.

[answers on page 50]

Mental state examination

246   Reciting the months of the year in reverse order is a test for short-term
       memory.

247   Reciting the months of the year in reverse order is a test for general
       knowledge.

248   Reciting the months of the year in reverse order is a test for long-term
       memory.

249   Reciting the months of the year in reverse order is usually impaired in
       agoraphobia.

250   Reciting the months of the year in reverse order is usually unimpaired
       in delirium tremens.

251   Reciting the months of the year in reverse order is a test for concentration.

252   Reciting the months of the year in reverse order can be impaired in
       generalized anxiety disorder.

253   Reciting the months of the year in reverse order varies depending upon
       the intellect level.

254   Reciting the months of the year in reverse order can be normal in the
       early stages of Alzheimer's disease.

255   Reciting the months of the year in reverse order can be impaired in
       depression.

[answers on page 51]

Physical/neurological examination

256   Clinical features of syringomyelia include loss of sensitivity to pain.

257   Clinical features of syringomyelia include loss of sensitivity to temperature.

258   Clinical features of syringomyelia include loss of sensitivity to touch.

259   Clinical features of syringomyelia include ulcers on the fingers.

260   Clinical features of syringomyelia include Bell's palsy.

[answers on page 51]

Answers and explanations

Basic sciences

Basic psychology

1   **True**   Schedules for reinforcement refer to the pattern or frequency with which a reinforcer is delivered as a consequence of behaviour.

2   **False**

3   **False**

4   **True**

5   **True**   Variable interval schedules are another type of reinforcement schedule.

6   **True**   Cognitive events refer to conscious, identifiable thoughts and images that are present in the stream of consciousness.

7   **False**

8   **False**

9   **True**   Cognitive processes refers to the processing of information.

10   **True**   Cognitive structures refers to attitudes or beliefs.

11   **False**   Primacy is given to thoughts and attitudes (cognitions).

12   **True**

13   **True**

14   **False**

15   **True**

16   **False**

17   **False**

18   **True**

19   **False**

20   **True**

21   **True**

22   **False**

23   **True**

24   **False**

25   **False**

26   **False**

27   **True**

28   **False**

29   **True**

30   **False**

31   **True**

32   **False**

33   **True**

Behavioural psychology

34 **True** Ellis' rational emotive therapy was influential in the development of cognitive–behavioural therapy.

35 **True** A schema is a particular set of attitudes and beliefs through which individuals appraise and interpret their environment, other people and themselves.

36 **True**

37 **False** Events tend to activate negative ways of thinking and precipitate depression in vulnerable individuals.

38 **True** The other components are: an individual's negative view of self and his or her negative interpretation of experiences.

39 **True** This principle is also known as Grandma's rule ('If you eat the spinach, you will get the dessert').

40 **False** It is the process by which a response that leads to removal of an aversive event is increased. A behaviour that enables a person or an animal to avoid or escape a punishing consequence is strengthened.

41 **True** Punishment reduces the probability that a response will occur.

Neuropsychology

42 **True** This is a visually presented test, where stimuli such as colours, shapes, etc., are presented and a relevant dimension needs to be identified. It measures abstract concept formation.

43 **False**

44 **False**

45 **False**

46 **True** It is over 90 per cent.

47 **True** This means that speech displays a profound lack of syntactic structure, i.e. impairments of the process involved in constructing the syntactic frame.

48 **True** There are marked impairments in semantic comprehension and in correct use of content and words, i.e. impairment of lexical access.

49 **True** It is associated with paraphasia, e.g. saying 'queen' as 'keen'.

50 **True** In extreme cases, patients are even unable to recognize their own faces in the mirror.

51 **False** It is loss of memory as a result of intense emotion or trauma. It is associated with 'fugue states'.

Human development

52 **False**

53 **False**

54 **False** It is affected by the state and temperament of both the caregiver and the child.

55 **True**

56 **False** It depends on building up a gradual relationship between the infant and caregiver over the first 6 months of life.

57   True
58   True
59   True
60   False
61   True
62   False
63   False

Psychopharmacology

General principles

64   True
65   True
66   False   Risperidone acts as an antagonist at central serotonergic S2 receptors.
67   False   It acts as an antagonist at both noradrenergic and histaminergic receptors.

Pharmacokinetics

68   False   In young adults it is about 20 hours, and in elderly people it is between 30 and 100 hours.
69   False   There is almost complete bioavailability with oral administration.
70   False   95 per cent is protein bound.
71   False   It is an active metabolite.
72   False   It reduces the rate and not the extent of absorption.
73   False   In therapeutic doses, benzodiazepines have little effect on the cardiovascular and respiratory systems, although, sometimes, they cause respiratory depression and reduce systolic blood pressure.
74   False
75   True   Chronic high-dose therapy may interfere with the dexamethasone suppression test.
76   True
77   True   Usually unchanged, although occasionally plasma cortisol may be reduced.

Pharmacodynamics

78   False   NMDA receptors are widely distributed in the brain and their activity is modified by magnesium ions.
79   False   Phencyclidine and ketamine block the NMDA-linked ion channels.
80   False   They are found in high concentrations in the hippocampus and cortex.
81   False   They may occur as a result of sudden release of glutamate.
82   True   Is associated with multi-infarct dementia.

Adverse drug reactions

83   False   It has less liability to produce extrapyramidal side effects.
84   False   The amount excreted in breast milk is too low to be harmful for the baby.
85   True   A significant amount of sulpiride is excreted in breast milk.
86   False
87   True
88   False
89   False   It may be associated with anorexia and subsequent weight loss.
90   False   It produces gastrointestinal disturbances, constipation and anorexia.
91   False
92   False
93   True
94   False
95   True
96   False
97   False   It is likely to cause pigmentation of the conjunctivae, cornea and eyelids. Pigmentary retinal degeneration or cataract can also occur.
98   True   It causes dilatation of pupils, affecting accommodation.

Psychopathology

Descriptive

99   False   Catatonia also occurs in organic and affective disorder.
100   False
101   True   In Mitmachen, the body can be put into any position without any resistance on the part of the patient, even though he or she has been instructed to resist all movements.
102   False   Gedankenlautwerden is the German term for audible thoughts that describe the patient's experiences of hearing his or her own thoughts said out loud. In French it is called 'echo de la pensée'.
103   False   The term was first introduced by Karl Kahlbaum.
104   True
105   True   It is one of the most striking features of obsessional personality. The person is rigid in his or her views and inflexible in his or her approach to problems.
106   True
107   False   This is a feature of antisocial personality disorder.
108   True   It is one of the most striking features of this disorder. The person finds it hard to weigh up advantages and disadvantages of new situations.
109   True
110   False   Visual hallucinations usually occur in organic brain and/or psychotic disorder.
111   True

112 False
113 True
114 False   The central feature of this syndrome is loss or impairment of function, which appears to be due to a physical cause but is in fact a manifestation of some underlying psychological conflict or need. The symptoms reduce unconscious anxiety.
115 False
116 False   The hysterical conversion symptoms are mediated via the peripheral nervous system.
117 True
118 False   The conversion symptoms usually confer some advantage on the patient by producing primary and secondary gains.
119 False   Return to work is unusual, and complete recovery is rare. In some patients, improvement does not occur even after the financial settlement.
120 True
121 True
122 False   These patients may have some difficulty with sleep.
123 False   The central feature is the seeking of financial compensation after sustaining a relatively trivial injury.
124 True
125 True
126 False
127 True
128 True
129 False
130 False
131 True
132 True   Hallucinogenic-type mushroom poisoning (*Psilocybe* and *Panaeolus* sp.) is characterized by mydriasis, nausea, vomiting and intense visual hallucinations.
133 False
134 False
135 False
136 True
137 False
138 True
139 True
140 False
141 False
142 True
143 True   Normal grief is characterized by three stages. The first stage consists of a lack of emotional reaction ('numbness') and a feeling of unreality that lasts for a few hours to several days. In the second stage, the person feels sad, weeps, sleeps badly and loses appetite. In the third stage, these symptoms subside gradually and the person accepts the new situation.
144 False

145 True

146 True

147 True

148 True

149 True   About half of the patients have episodes of uncontrollable overeating during which they may eat large amounts of food that they would usually avoid.

150 False

151 False

152 True   Bulimia refers to episodes of uncontrolled excessive eating.

153 True   Some depressed patients eat more and therefore gain weight. It seems as if eating brings temporary relief to their distressing feelings.

154 True

155 False   It is a sign of anorexia nervosa.

156 False

157 True

158 True

159 True

160 True   They are often associated with sleepwalking.

161 True

162 False   Night terrors occur in stages III and IV of sleep, which are associated with low-frequency delta and theta rhythm. Alpha rhythm occurs between 8 and 13 Hz.

163 False

164 True

165 False

166 False

167 True

168 False

169 True

Psychodynamic

170 False   Paranosic means primary advantage derived from an illness, i.e. primary gain. The question refers to a secondary gain.

171 True

172 True

173 False   It refers to secondary gain.

174 True

175 True

176 False   Transference is not interpreted in supportive psychotherapy.

177 False   Transference is not a response to countertransference or vice versa. Countertransference is the analyst's own strong feeling towards the patient.

178 False

179 True

180 **False**   The patient with obsessive–compulsive disorder uses regression, intellectualization and other ego defence mechanisms.

181 **True**

182 **False**

183 **True**

184 **True**

185 **True**   Id is a completely unconscious intrapsychic agency that is only interested in discharging tension.

186 **True**   The conscious aspect of the ego is the executive organ of the psyche, responsible for decision making and integration of perceptual data. The unconscious aspect of the ego contains the defence mechanisms.

187 **True**

188 **True**   For most part, the superego is unconscious, but aspects of it are certainly conscious. The conscious level of functioning involves 'secondary processes' which are logical, rational and geared to meeting the demands of the real world.

189 **True**

190 **True**   This is a special method of psychotherapy developed by Freud, dealing particularly with transference.

191 **False**   Dynamic psychotherapy is concerned with the largely unconsciously derived and transferred feelings and attitudes, which the patient invests in the analyst.

192 **True**

193 **False**

194 **False**   It includes analysis of unconscious conflicts, deficits and distortions of intrapsychic structures and internal object relations.

195 **True**   The id represents all the inherited biological and constitutional features of the individuals including instincts and basic drives.

196 **False**   The ego is reality oriented and finds acceptable and appropriate ways of satisfying the demands of the id and superego.

197 **True**

198 **True**

199 **False**   The id operates according to the hedonistic pleasure principle in that it avoids being frustrated and seeks immediate gratification regardless of consequences.

200 **True**

201 **False**

202 **True**

203 **True**

204 **True**   In brief focal dynamic psychotherapy, five to 20 sessions might be allocated depending on the complexity of the problems. The therapist emphasizes that the patient will be helped to find his or her own solutions to the problems.

Clinical theory and skills

Aetiology

205 **True**

206 **False** Papilloedema (swelling of the optic disc due to raised intracranial pressure) is usually bilateral and produces enlargement of the blind spot without loss of acuity. The causes of papilloedema include posterior uveitis, posterior scleritis, optic neuritis, anterior ischaemic optic neuropathy, optic nerve sheath meningioma, sarcoidosis, leukaemia and lymphoma.

207 **True**

208 **True**

209 **False**

210 **False**

211 **False**

212 **True**

213 **True**

214 **True**

Classification/diagnosis

215 **True**

216 **False** The aetiology of Wilson's disease is known but it is not classified as a psychiatric disorder.

217 **True**

218 **False** Aetiology of Alzheimer's disease is unknown.

219 **False** Aetiology of Briquet's syndrome is unknown.

220 **False** Most diagnoses are dependent on multiple symptoms rather than single symptoms.

221 **True**

222 **True**

223 **False** There are few validating criteria such as laboratory tests.

224 **False** When inferences need to be drawn as in determining psychodynamic defence mechanisms, the reliability tends to be poor.

225 **False** Alcohol abuse is in the same group as abuse of other substances.

226 **False** All mood disorders have been brought under the same grouping as opposed to ICD-9 in which depression occurred in 13 different categories.

227 **False**

228 **True**

229 **False**

History taking/interviewing

230 **True** Although the mental state examination is largely concerned with what the patient says much can also be learned from observing his or her general appearance, behaviour, mood, posture, movements, etc.

231 **True**

232 **False**   This indicates the patient's subjective feelings.
233 **True**
234 **True**
235 **False**   In reflection, although a part of what the patient has said is repeated, it is not necessarily an exact repetition of what the patient said.
236 **False**   Direct questions are used to gather specific information.
237 **False**   The true answer is clarification.
238 **False**   Silence is an important component of interviewing.
239 **False**   Recapitulation, i.e. summation, would be logical only towards the end of the interview.
240 **True**
241 **True**
242 **False**
243 **False**   Changing the topic (switching) or explaining away things as if they are expected (normalization) as well as improper reassurances, frequently leads to inadequate information being elicited.
244 **True**
245 **True**

Mental state examination

246 **False**   It is a test of concentration.
247 **False**
248 **False**
249 **False**
250 **False**
251 **True**
252 **True**
253 **True**
254 **True**
255 **True**

Physical/neurological examination

256 **True**   In the early stages, there is dissociated sensory loss.
257 **True**
258 **False**   Sensitivity to touch is retained because the posterior column is preserved.
259 **True**   The ulcers arise from painless cuts and burns.
260 **False**

PAPER 2 ISQs

Questions

Basic sciences

Basic psychology

1   Self-psychology is derived from the seminal writings of Kernberg.

2   Self-psychology stresses how external relationships help maintain self-esteem and self-cohesion.

3   Self-psychology deals with mirror-transference and idealizing-transference.

4   Self-psychology is of no use in treating narcissistic patients.

5   Self-psychology is the same as object relations theory.

6   As regards schedules of reinforcement, a smooth pattern of behaviour is found with a variable-ratio schedule.

7   As regards schedules of reinforcement, the rate of response decreases following reinforcement in a fixed-ratio schedule.

8   As regards schedules of reinforcement, in a variable-ratio schedule the rate of response tends to be rapid.

9   As regards schedules of reinforcement, 'scalloping' occurs in a fixed-interval schedule.

10 As regards schedules of reinforcement, in a fixed-interval schedule the number of responses increases in inverse proportion to the duration of the interval.

11 The object relations theory is fundamentally similar to ego psychology.

12 As regards object relations theory, Melanie Klein is usually considered as the founder of the object relations movement.

13 The object relations theory encompasses the transformation of interpersonal relationships into internalized representations of relationships.

14 As regards object relations theory, Fairburn coined the term 'good enough mothering'.

15 As regards object relations theory, Melanie Klein described 'paranoid and depressive positions'.

16   Mowerer's two-step conditioning process was hypothesized to explain obsessions.

17   Mowerer's two-step conditioning process forms the basis for systematic desensitization.

18   In Mowerer's two-step conditioning process, the first step refers to the development of fears in early childhood.

19   Mowerer's two-step conditioning uses concepts of both classical and operant conditioning.

20   In Mowerer's two-step conditioning process, the second step refers to the reinforcing aspect of avoidance.

[answers on page 66]

Behavioural psychology

21   The cognitive model of anxiety states that events are responsible for anxiety.

22   The cognitive model of anxiety states that people's interpretation of events is responsible for anxiety.

23   The cognitive model of anxiety states that interpretation of perceived loss is responsible for anxiety.

24   The cognitive model of anxiety states that cognitions relate to perceived danger.

25   The cognitive model of anxiety states that the patient's responses are appropriate to the situations in which they occur.

26   Cognitive–behavioural aspects of depression include object loss.

27   Cognitive–behavioural aspects of depression include denial.

28   Cognitive–behavioural aspects of depression include learned helplessness.

29   Cognitive–behavioural aspects of depression include diminished social skills.

30   Cognitive–behavioural aspects of depression include scapegoating.

31   Learned helplessness was first described by Seligman.

32   Learned helplessness has been used in experiments with animals.

33   Learned helplessness is frequently seen in depression.

34   Learned helplessness occurs when reward is no longer contingent on the desired behaviour.

35   Learned helplessness is commonly associated with social phobia.

36   In aversive conditioning, an organism changes its behaviour to avoid a painful stimulus.

37   Adventitious reinforcement plays a role in the pathogenesis of phobias.

[answers on page 66]

Neuropsychology

38   Wechsler's Adult Intelligence Scale–Revised assesses constructional ability.

39   The Rey–Osterreith Figure Test assesses immediate and delayed recall of complex spatial material.

40   Stroop's Test is a general organic screening procedure.

41   The Category Test is a general organic screening procedure.

42   The Trail Making Test is a specific test for detecting brain damage.

43   The Wisconsin Card Sorting Test is used to detect disturbance of reasoning, abstraction and logical analysis.

44   In phobias, attenuation of response to unconditioned stimuli usually occurs.

45   The psychometric approach is atheoretical and lacks a driving theory of cognition.

46   Wechsler's Memory Scale–Revised is a diagnostic test that does not discriminate memory disturbance of organic and psychogenic origin.

47   Rennick's Repeatable Battery is sensitive to organic impairment and small but definable changes over time.

48   Stroop's Color-Word Inference Test is sensitive to brain damage.

49   Positron emission tomography (PET) scanning is useful in determining cerebral dominance for language.

[answers on page 67]

Human development

50   Jean Piaget is best known for his theories on the types of intrapsychic defence mechanism.

51   Jean Piaget is best known for his theories on the meanings of symbols.

52   According to Bowlby, primary attachments may be formed through middle childhood.

53   According to Bowlby, the primary attachment figure is not necessarily the biological mother.

54   According to Bowlby, infants are likely to form attachments to those children and adults with whom they come into daily contact.

55   The child's first attachment relationship has to be formed in the first few hours of life to ensure the subsequent socioeconomic wellbeing of the child.

56   Secondary attachments may, for some children, give 'protection' against any possible effects of the absence of a secure attachment to the primary caregiver.

57   According to Piaget's theory of cognitive development, syncretic reasoning is a feature of preoperational stage.

58   According to Piaget's theory of cognitive development, transductive reasoning is a feature of the sensorimotor stage.

59   According to Piaget's theory of cognitive development, preoperational children have difficulty with reversibility.

60   According to Piaget's theory of cognitive development, hypothetico-deductive reasoning emerges during the concrete operational stage.

61   According to Piaget's theory of cognitive development, the child is able to learn to classify items into hierarchies and sort items according to several dimensions or features during the concrete operational stage.

[answers on page 68]

Psychopharmacology

Pharmacokinetics

62   The term 'therapeutic index' refers to the ratio of maximum tolerated concentration (MTC) and minimum effective concentration (MEC).

63   With regard to the pharmacokinetics of benzodiazepines, the long-acting agents have a long elimination half-life.

64   With regard to the pharmacokinetics of benzodiazepines, the short-acting agents have a small distribution volume.

65   With regard to pharmacokinetics of benzodiazepines, the long-acting agents have no active metabolites.

66   With regard to the pharmacokinetics of benzodiazepines, the short-acting agents have minimum accumulation.

67   With regard to the pharmacokinetics of benzodiazepines, anxiolytic drugs have a half-life of 12 hours.

68   With reference to pharmacokinetics, drugs with large distribution volumes will invariably reach the transcellular regions such as the brain and fetus.

69   With reference to pharmacokinetics, phenylbutazone has a similar volume of distribution to plasma volume.

70   With reference to pharmacokinetics, haloperidol possesses a volume of distribution greater than 2 L/kg.

71   With reference to pharmacokinetics, dopamine is able to cross the blood–brain barrier.

[answers on page 68]

Pharmacodynamics

72   With reference to neurotransmitters, Dale's law states that for each neurone, the same neurotransmitter is released at all its synapses.

73   According to current scientific knowledge, a neurotransmitter must be present in a nerve terminal and in the vicinity of the area of the brain where it is thought to act.

74   With reference to neurotransmitters, a neurotransmitter is released from the nerve terminal following nerve stimulation.

75   With reference to neurotransmitters, a neurotransmitter activates a post-synaptic receptor site following its release.

76   With reference to neurotransmitters, enzymes concerned in the synthesis and metabolism of a neurotransmitter should be present in the nerve ending.

77   With regard to the process of 'depolarization' in a neurone, it opens up potassium channels.

78   With regard to the process of 'depolarization' in a neurone, closing of sodium channels causes the falling phase of the action potential.

79   With regard to the physiology of a neurone, all nerve cells action potentials are followed by transient hyperpolarization.

80   With reference to 'depolarization' in a neurone, during the refractory period, it is impossible to trigger an action potential.

81   All excitatory neurotransmitters produce excitatory post-synaptic potentials.

[answers on page 68]

Adverse drug reactions

82   Fine tremors are a frequent side effect of tricyclic antidepressant drugs.

83   Insomnia is a common side effect of tricyclic antidepressant drugs.

84   Nausea is a frequent side effect of tricyclic antidepressant drugs.

85   Constipation is a common side effect of tricyclic antidepressant drugs.

86   Skin rash is a side effect of tricyclic antidepressant drugs.

87   Vomiting is a frequent side effect of selective serotonin reuptake inhibitor drugs in therapeutic doses.

88   Headache is a common side effect of selective serotonin reuptake inhibitor drugs in therapeutic doses.

89   Drowsiness is a frequent side effect of selective serotonin reuptake inhibitor drugs in therapeutic doses.

90   Diarrhoea is a frequent side effect of selective serotonin reuptake inhibitor drugs in therapeutic doses.

91   As regards treatment with neuroleptic drugs, akathisia usually occurs in the first 7 days of treatment.

92   As regards treatment with neuroleptic drugs, elderly females are more prone to extrapyramidal side effects.

93   As regards treatment with neuroleptic drugs, young males are prone to tardive dyskinesia.

94   As regards treatment with neuroleptic drugs, akathisia occurs less frequently than dystonia.

95   As regards treatment with neuroleptic drugs, concomitant antiparkinsonian drug should not be prescribed routinely.

96   Carbamazepine is contraindicated in patients with hepatic failure.

97   Chlorpromazine is contraindicated in patients with hepatic failure.

98   Fluvoxamine is contraindicated in patients with hepatic failure.

99   Paroxetine is contraindicated in patients with hepatic failure.

100   Lofepramine is contraindicated in patients with hepatic failure.

[answers on page 68]

Psychopathology

Descriptive

101   Somatic manifestations of psychiatric disorders occur more commonly in elderly patients.

102   Somatic manifestations of psychiatric disorders occur more commonly in children than adults.

103   Somatic manifestations of psychiatric disorders occur more commonly in patients from higher social classes than those from lower social classes.

104   Somatic manifestations of psychiatric disorders occur more commonly in people from Eastern countries than in people from Western countries.

105   The origins of somatic manifestations of psychiatric disorders are considered to be culturally determined.

106   Hyperphagia characteristically occurs in the Klüver–Bucy syndrome.

107   Hyperphagia characteristically occurs in the Kleine–Levin syndrome.

108   Hyperphagia characteristically occurs in anorexia nervosa.

109   Hyperphagia characteristically occurs in bulimia nervosa.

110   Hyperphagia characteristically occurs in bipolar affective disorder.

111   Catatonic phenomena include posturing.

112   Catatonic phenomena include Lhermitte's sign.

113   Catatonic phenomena include negativism.

114   Catatonic phenomena include command automatism.

115   Catatonic phenomena include periods of excitement.

116   The depersonalization–derealization syndrome is significantly associated with 'near-death' experiences.

117   The depersonalization–derealization syndrome is significantly associated with phobic disorders.

118   The depersonalization–derealization syndrome is significantly associated with obsessive–compulsive disorder.

119   The depersonalization–derealization syndrome is significantly associated with sensory deprivation.

120   The depersonalization–derealization syndrome is significantly associated with depression.

121   Disturbances regarding the passage of time occur in patients with major depression.

122   Disturbances regarding the passage of time occur in patients with chronic fatigue syndrome.

123   Disturbances regarding the passage of time occur in patients suffering from depersonalization.

124   Disturbances regarding the passage of time occur in patients intoxicated with LSD.

125   Disturbances regarding the passage of time occur in patients suffering from mania.

126   Depersonalization is associated with increased anxiety.

127   Depersonalization is usually associated with serialization.

128   Depersonalization usually lasts for a short period in normal people.

129   Depersonalization is a characteristic feature of depression.

130   Depersonalization is frequently associated with panic attacks.

131   Partial amnesia on recovery is a characteristic feature of clouding of consciousness.

132   Disorientation with regard to time, place and person is a characteristic feature of clouding of consciousness.

133   Visual hallucinations are a characteristic feature of clouding of consciousness.

134   Perplexed mood is a characteristic feature of clouding of consciousness.

135   Restlessness is a characteristic feature of clouding of consciousness.

136   Echolalia is a characteristic feature of catatonia.

137   Cataplexy is a characteristic feature of catatonia.

138   Psychological pillow is a characteristic feature of catatonia.

139   Stereotypies are characteristic features of catatonia.

140   Echopraxia is a characteristic feature of catatonia.

141   Hypochondriacal delusions are a recognized feature in schizophrenia.

142   Hypochondriacal delusions are a recognized feature in illness phobia.

143   Hypochondriacal delusions are a recognized feature in social phobia.

144   Hypochondriacal delusions are a recognized feature in severe depression.

145   Hypochondriacal delusions are a recognized feature in somatoform disorders.

146   Anhedonia is associated with long-term use of phenobarbital.

147   Anhedonia can be detected by a depression rating scale.

148   Anhedonia refers to the loss of pleasure in pastimes.

149   Anhedonia was first described by Anna Freud.

150   Anhedonia is a diagnostic feature of major depression.

151   A hallucination is defined as misperception or misinterpretation of real external stimuli.

152   Hallucinations include actual sense deception but not distortion of a real perception.

153   An autoscopy is a form of visual hallucination.

154   Deaf people do not experience auditory hallucinations.

[answers on page 69]

Dynamic

155   In phobias, the main defence mechanism is similar to that found in conversion disorder.

156   In phobias, repression is the first defence mechanism employed by patients.

157   Different ego defence mechanisms operate in patients suffering from agoraphobia and social phobia.

158   Oedipal complex is an unconscious conflict experienced by patients with phobias.

159   Isolation and undoing are important defence mechanisms operating in patients suffering from social phobia.

160   Displacement is a neurotic defence mechanism.

161   Rationalization is a primitive defence mechanism.

162   Somatization is a neurotic defence mechanism.

163   Projection is a neurotic defence mechanism.

164   Splitting is a primitive defence mechanism.

165   Sigmund Freud is considered as the father of ego psychology.

166   Sigmund Freud put forward id, ego and superego as a topographical model of the mind.

167   Sigmund Freud described the Oedipus complex in girls and the Electra complex in boys.

168   Sigmund Freud considered the id to be a completely unconscious intrapsychic conflict.

169   Sigmund Freud described the oral and anal stages as the first two stages of psychosexual development.

170   According to psychodynamic theories, depression is linked to the depressive position as described by Melanie Klein.

171   According to psychodynamic theories, depression occurs as a result of introjection of a lost object.

172   According to psychodynamic theories, aggression is considered pivotal to the understanding of depression as described by Bibring.

173   According to psychodynamic theories, depression is similar to the process of mourning.

174   According to psychodynamic theories of depression, the patient psychogenetically regresses to the oral stage of psychosexual development.

175   Transference may play a role in accusatory behaviour.

176   Regression results in the patient's feelings and thinking as though he or she were a child, which may in turn contribute to impulsivity and increased transference feelings.

177   Sublimation is the channelling of unacceptable impulses into acceptable and creative channels.

178   Dream becomes somewhat more rational by secondary process than secondary revision.

179   Suppression and repression are synonymous in terms of defence mechanisms.

[answers on page 71]

Clinical theory and skills

Aetiology

180   Uraemia is a reversible cause of cognitive impairment.

181   Parkinson's disease is a reversible cause of cognitive impairment.

182   Depression is a reversible cause of cognitive impairment.

183   Alcohol abuse is a reversible cause of cognitive impairment.

184   Benzodiazepines cause reversible cognitive impairment.

185   As regards self-inflicted harm in elderly people, men are more often involved than women.

186   As regards self-inflicted harm in elderly people, it is often precipitated by financial stress.

187   As regards self-inflicted harm in elderly people, the associated mortality is lower than in the younger age group.

188   Self-inflicted harm in elderly people is often associated with a significant mental disorder.

189   As regards self-inflicted harm in elderly people, bereavement is considered to be an important precipitating factor.

[answers on page 72]

Classification/diagnosis

190   In comparison with Diagnostic and Statistical Manual (DSM)-IV, the International Classification of Diseases (ICD)-10 includes post-psychotic depression under affective disorders.

191   In comparison with DSM-IV, ICD-10 has an extensive classification of short-lived psychotic disorders.

192   In comparison with DSM-IV, ICD-10 includes schizotypal disorder under schizophrenia.

193   In comparison with DSM-IV, ICD-10 extends the age of onset of autism to 48 months.

194   In comparison with DSM-IV, ICD-10 uses narcissistic personality as an inclusion term for passive–aggressive personality disorder.

195   ICD-10 is essentially a multi-axial classification.

196   ICD-10 is mainly a classification system of adult psychiatric disorders.

197   ICD-10 provides practical guidance regarding psychiatric diagnosis.

198   ICD-10 does not use the word 'hysteria' at all in the text.

199   ICD-10 contains only mental and behavioural disorders.

200   The ICD-10 was developed by the World Health Organization.

201   The ICD-10 is extensively used in Europe.

202   The ICD-10 uses separate coding for severity.

203   The ICD-10 is applicable only to hospitalized patients.

204   With regards to the ICD-10, it is the basis of statistical information for the National Health Service in the UK.

[answers on page 72]

History taking/interviewing

205   Psychosexual history in a severely depressed, married patient should include repeated masturbation.

206   Psychosexual history in a severely depressed, married patient should include recent change in sexual behaviour.

207   Psychosexual history in a severely depressed, married patient should include a number of previous sexual partners.

208   Psychosexual history in a severely depressed, married patient should include recent change in sexual desire.

209   Psychosexual history in a severely depressed, married patient should include latent homosexuality.

210   A good diagnostic interviewing technique is maintaining constant eye-to-eye contact with the patient.

211   A good diagnostic interviewing technique is to directly ask the patient about his or her feelings.

212   A good diagnostic interviewing technique is avoiding uncomfortable silences during the interview.

213   A good diagnostic interviewing technique is to adjourn questions about alcohol use until a follow-up interview.

214   A good diagnostic interviewing technique is to avoid taking notes during the interview.

215   Inability to sit during an interview is a diagnostic feature of hypomania.

216   Inability to sit during an interview occurs in absence of a mental illness.

217   Inability to sit during an interview does not occur in patients with Alzheimer's disease.

218   Inability to sit during an interview is a characteristic feature of patients suffering from generalized anxiety disorder.

219   Inability to sit during an interview may be due to dystonia.

220   A clarifying statement is used to avoid taking at face value certain words expressed by the patient.

221   A self-relevant statement should only be used sparingly with new patients.

222   During an interview, it is important to give non-verbal cues of disapproval if the patient makes one feel angry.

[answers on page 72]

Mental state examination

223   Valid tests of orientation in a delirious patient include giving correct date of birth.

224   Valid tests of orientation in a delirious patient include the ability to perform mental arithmetic.

225   Valid tests of orientation in a delirious patient include an awareness of the role of the interviewer.

226   Valid tests of orientation in a delirious patient include a correct awareness of passage of time.

227   Valid tests of orientation in a delirious patient include giving the correct address.

228   When testing short-term memory, a 5-minute interval between presenting information and asking for its recall is sufficient.

229   In a mental state examination, if the serial sevens test cannot be performed reliably, the digit span test will be a reliable test of short-term memory.

230   In a mental state examination, recalling the months of the year in reverse order is a satisfactory substitution for the serial sevens test.

231   In a mental state examination, misidentification of date with an error of 2 days is a sensitive indicator of disorientation.

232   As regards mental state examination, poor recall of the Babcock sentence is a reliable indicator of the presence of organic brain disorder.

233   Depressed mood in a patient may be suggested by a drooping of the angle of the mouth.

234   Depressed mood in a patient may be suggested by a raised medial aspect of the eyebrow.

235   The patient talking with a soft voice may be suggestive of depressed mood in that patient.

236   A patient using only limited vocabulary may be suggestive of depressed mood in that patient.

237   Depressed mood in a patient may be suggested by the patient's avoidance of eye-to-eye contact.

238   Enduring cognitive deficits are less severe in bipolar affective disorder than in schizophrenia.

239   Cognitive impairment in schizophrenia is global and not selective.

240   Cognitive impairment in schizophrenia is independent of the clinical state of the patient.

[answers on page 73]

Physical/neurological examination

241   Clinical features of Bell's palsy include facial paralysis.

242   Clinical features of Bell's palsy include ptosis of eyelid.

243   Clinical features of Bell's palsy include drooling of saliva from the corner of the mouth.

244   Clinical features of Bell's palsy include hyperacusis.

245 Clinical features of Bell's palsy include trigeminal neuralgia.

246 A characteristic feature of pseudobulbar palsy is exaggerated jaw jerk.

247 A characteristic feature of pseudobulbar palsy is emotional lability.

248 A characteristic feature of pseudobulbar palsy is wasting of the tongue.

249 Characteristic features of pseudobulbar palsy include fasciculations of facial muscles.

250 A characteristic feature of pseudobulbar palsy is dysphonia.

251 Significant memory loss occurs with temporal lobe lesions.

252 Significant memory loss occurs with lesions of the uncus.

253 Significant memory loss occurs with lesions in the amygdala.

254 Significant memory loss occurs with microscopic haemorrhages in the mammillary bodies.

255 Significant memory loss occurs with left parietal lobe lesions.

256 Absent knee and ankle jerks are a characteristic feature of Huntington's chorea.

257 Absent knee and ankle jerks are a characteristic feature of Punch-drunk syndrome.

258 Absent knee and ankle jerks are a characteristic feature of Guillain–Barré syndrome.

259 Absent knee and ankle jerks are a characteristic feature of motor neurone disease.

260 Absent knee and ankle jerks are characteristically present in Alzheimer's disease.

[answers on page 74]

Answers and explanations

Basic sciences

Basic psychology

1   **False**   Self-psychology is derived from the seminal writings of Heinz Kohut. It stresses how external relationships maintain self-esteem and self-cohesion.
2   **True**
3   **True**
4   **False**   It is of particular help while treating narcissistic patients.
5   **False**   Object relations theory is derived from the work of Melanie Klein, Fairburn, Winnicott and Balint.
6   **False**   Due to the variability in responses with fixed schedules, variable schedules are used to obtain smooth patterns of responding.
7   **True**
8   **True**
9   **True**   'Scalloping' refers to the increase in responses that occur as the time for reinforcement draws nearer.
10   **True**
11   **False**   Object relations theory differs from ego-psychology in two important ways: (i) it considers drives as secondary and not primary and (ii) it has compressed the development timetable of classical theory into the first year of life.
12   **True**
13   **True**
14   **False**   Winnicott coined the phrase 'good enough mothering'.
15   **True**
16   **False**   The two-step conditioning process was hypothesized to underlie the development of fear and by analogy the phobic disorder.
17   **False**
18   **False**   The first step involves the pairing of a stimulus situation with fear (classical conditioning).
19   **True**
20   **True**   The second step involves reinforcing avoidance of the now feared situation by anxiety reduction (operant conditioning).

Behavioural psychology

21   **False**   In the cognitive model, it is not the events *per se* but people's expectations and interpretations that are responsible for negative emotions.
22   **True**
23   **False**   Perceived loss is important in depression.
24   **True**

25   **False**   The patient's responses are considered inappropriate and out of proportion to the perceived danger.
26   **False**
27   **False**
28   **True**
29   **True**
30   **False**   This is a phenomenon observed in group psychotherapy where some patients may become 'scapegoated' because of their more primitive psychopathology and their greater tendency to express affect in a direct manner.
31   **True**   In 1975, Seligman suggested that depression developed when reward or punishment is no longer clearly contingent upon the actions of the organism.
32   **True**
33   **False**   Learned helplessness is not a symptom of depression.
34   **True**
35   **False**
36   **True**
37   **False**

Neuropsychology

38   **True**
39   **True**
40   **True**
41   **True**
42   **False**   It is a general organic screening procedure.
43   **True**
44   **False**   It does not occur.
45   **True**
46   **False**   It provides a broad assessment of predominantly short-term memory and learning.
47   **True**
48   **True**
49   **True**

Human development

50   **False**
51   **False**
52   **True**
53   **True**
54   **True**
55   **False**
56   **True**
57   **True**
58   **False**

59 True
60 False
61 True

Psychopharmacology

Pharmacokinetics

62 **True**
63 **True**
64 **False** They have a large distribution volume.
65 **False**
66 **True**
67 **False** Anxiolytics tend to have a half-life in the region of 40–100 hours. Hypnotics have a half-life of 8–12 hours.
68 **True**
69 **True** It reflects the drug's strong affinity for plasma proteins.
70 **True**
71 **False**

Pharmacodynamics

72 **True** Dale's law applies only to the presynaptic effects.
73 **True**
74 **True** It is generally a calcium-dependent process.
75 **True**
76 **True** They should be present in the proximity of the nerve endings.
77 **False** Sodium channels open up increasing the sodium ion influx into the cell and producing the rising phase of the action potential.
78 **True** Because the influx of sodium ions is reduced.
79 **False** This happens in most nerve cells but not all.
80 **False** This is possible if the stimulus is stronger than normal.
81 **True** They last for approximately 5 ms.

Adverse drug reactions

82 **True**
83 **False**
84 **True**
85 **True**
86 **True** Other side effects include dry mouth, sedation, blurred vision and sweating.
87 **True**
88 **True**
89 **True**
90 **True** Other common side effects include nausea, tremors, insomnia, agitation and increased sweating.

91 **True** It is characterized by motor restlessness, a subjective feeling of tension, and inability to tolerate inactivity which gives rise to restless movements.

92 **True**

93 **False** Tardive dyskinesia is more common among women, elderly patients and patients who have diffuse brain pathology. In half of the cases, it appears when the drugs are stopped.

94 **False** Acute dystonia occurs in 2–10 per cent of patients treated with typical antipsychotics.

95 **True** Routine administration of such drugs is not justified as not all patients are affected. Tardive dyskinesia may be unmasked or worsened by them. These drugs are abused for their mood-altering effects.

96 **False**

97 **False**

98 **False**

99 **False** The dose should be reduced.

100 **True**

Psychopathology

Descriptive

101 **True**

102 **True**

103 **False**

104 **True**

105 **True** Mental disorders presenting physical symptoms are heterogeneous and difficult to classify. It is probable that most symptoms arise in part from the misinterpretation of normal bodily sensations and trivial physical complaints, distress being expressed in bodily rather than in psychological terms.

106 **True**

107 **True**

108 **False**

109 **True**

110 **False**

111 **True**

112 **False**

113 **True**

114 **True**

115 **True**

116 **True**

117 **True**

118 **False**

119 **True**

120 **True**   Depersonalization and derealization are experienced quite commonly as transient phenomena by healthy adults and children, especially when tired. The experience usually begins abruptly and in normal people seldom lasts more than a few minutes. The symptoms may occur after sleep deprivation.

121 **True**

122 **True**

123 **True**

124 **True**

125 **True**   It is also well known that the experience of the passage of time varies in normal circumstances. When a person is happy or engrossed, time seems to pass very fast; when they are feeling sad, bored or idle, it drags.

126 **True**

127 **True**

128 **True**

129 **False**

130 **True**   Depersonalization is particularly associated with generalized and phobic anxiety disorders, depression, schizophrenia and sensory deprivation.

131 **False**   Amnesia may occur on recovery. The patients are likely to show memory disturbances and disorientation while having clouded consciousness.

132 **True**

133 **False**   Clouding of consciousness denotes the mildest stage of impairment of consciousness on a continuum from full alertness and awareness to coma.

134 **True**

135 **True**

136 **True**   Echolalia means that the patient refers to words or parts of sentences that are spoken to him or her in his or her presence.

137 **False**   Cataplexy refers to sudden temporary episodes of paralysis with loss of muscle tone. It is one of the characteristic features of narcolepsy.

138 **True**   Psychological pillow refers to a condition in which the patient's head is maintained a few inches above the bed for a sustained period of time which may go on for hours.

139 **True**   Stereotypy refers to persistent repetition of gestures or movements that do not appear to be goal-directed.

140 **True**   Echopraxia refers to the patient's imitation of the interviewer's every action.

141 **True**

142 **False**

143 **False**

144 **True**

145 **False**   Differentiation from hypochondriacal delusions usually depends upon close acquaintance with the patient. Although the beliefs are longstanding and appear to be firmly held, the degree of conviction is usually susceptible.

146 **True**

147 **True**

148 **True**

149 **False**

150 **True**   Anhedonia means total inability to enjoy anything in life or even get the accustomed satisfaction from usual leisure activities.

151 **False**

152 **True**

153 **True**

154 **False**

Dynamic

155 **False**   The main defence mechanism employed in phobias is displacement, whereas conversion is the main defence mechanism in conversion disorders.

156 **True**

157 **False**   In both disorders, the defence mechanisms involved are the same, i.e. repression, displacement and avoidance.

158 **True**

159 **False**   The defence mechanisms that are important for obsessive–compulsive disorder are isolation and undoing and not for social phobia.

160 **True**

161 **False**   It is a neurotic defence mechanism.

162 **True**

163 **False**   It is a primitive defence mechanism.

164 **True**

165 **True**

166 **False**   Id, ego and superego are a structural model of the mind.

167 **False**   Freud described the Oedipus complex in boys and the Electra complex in girls.

168 **True**

169 **True**

170 **True**

171 **True**

172 **False**   Bibring believed that depression was a primary affective state unrelated to aggression turned inwards.

173 **True**   In psychoanalytic understanding, depression is similar to melancholia and mourning. Freud suggested that the causes of mourning and depression might be similar, e.g. mourning results from loss by death and depression results from actual loss or loss of 'some abstraction'.

174 **True**

175 **True**

176 **True**

177 **True**

178 **True**

179 **False**

Clinical theory and skills

Aetiology

180 **True**
181 **False**
182 **True**
183 **False**
184 **True**
185 **True**
186 **False**
187 **False**
188 **True**
189 **True**

Classification/diagnosis

190 **False**   Post-psychotic depression is included under schizophrenia.
191 **True**
192 **True**
193 **False**
194 **False**   Neither narcissistic nor passive–aggressive personality disorder has been included in ICD-10.
195 **False**   There is a multi-axial presentation in Chapter V (F) of ICD-10, but it is not used in the main classification.
196 **False**   ICD-10 covers mental disorders occurring in all age groups.
197 **True**
198 **False**   ICD-10 includes the word 'hysteria' in the chapter on neurotic, stress-related and somatoform disorders (F40 to F48). However, hysterical disorders are referred to as dissociative conversion disorders.
199 **False**   Only chapter V (F) refers to mental disorders.
200 **True**   ICD-10 is designed to be a central (core) classification for a family of diseases and related classifications. Chapter V refers to mental and behavioural disorders.
201 **True**
202 **False**   Distinguishing between different grades of severity remains a problem. In mood disorders, three grades of disorders, mild, moderate and severe have been specified. There is a separate coding for somatic, psychotic or mixed symptoms in certain diagnostic categories.
203 **False**   ICD-10 is considered suitable for both primary and secondary healthcare.
204 **True**

History taking/interviewing

205 **False**
206 **True**
207 **False**

208 **True**

209 **False**

210 **False**

211 **True**   The interview should start by giving the patient free rein to describe his or her problems as he or she sees them. The initial questions should be as wide and open-ended as possible.

212 **False**

213 **False**

214 **False**   Record the patient's replies to key questions and any striking or unusual remarks verbatim.

215 **True**   Hypomanic patients are usually overactive and restless.

216 **True**

217 **False**

218 **False**   Anxious patients are often tremulous and restless.

219 **False**   Patients on antipsychotic drugs experience dystonia and akathisia. Akathisia is an unpleasant feeling of physical restlessness and a need to move, leading to an inability to keep still.

220 **True**

221 **True**

222 **False**

Mental state examination

223 **False**   This is a test of long-term memory.

224 **False**

225 **True**

226 **True**

227 **False**   This is a test of long-term memory.

228 **True**

229 **False**   Serial sevens is a test of concentration and not short-term memory.

230 **True**

231 **False**

232 **False**   Three repetitions of such a sentence are usually enough for correct immediate reproduction by a healthy young person. However, this test does not satisfactorily discriminate patients with organic brain disorder from patients with depressive disorder or even from healthy young people.

233 **True**

234 **True**

235 **True**

236 **True**

237 **True**   Other features include vertical furrows on the brow, and hunched shoulders with sitting or leaning forward.

238 **True**

239 **True**

240 **True**

Physical/neurological examination

241 **True** Bell's palsy is a common disorder caused by neuritis (possibly viral in origin) of the facial nerve. Facial paralysis is usually complete on the affected side.

242 **True** The patient is unable to raise the eyebrow, close the eye or retract the lip.

243 **True**

244 **True**

245 **False**

246 **True**

247 **True**

248 **True** The tongue is contracted and spastic. It cannot be moved rapidly from side to side.

249 **True**

250 **False** The patient experiences difficulty in swallowing, chewing, coughing, breathing and talking (dysarthria).

251 **True**

252 **True**

253 **True**

254 **True**

255 **False** Parietal lobe syndrome is characterized by visuo-spatial difficulties, such as constructional apraxia and visuo-spatial agnosia, topographical disorientation, visual inattention, sensory jacksonian fits and cortical sensory loss.

256 **False**

257 **False** Punch-drunk syndrome is characterized by cerebellar, pyramidal and extra-pyramidal signs, as well as intellectual deterioration.

258 **True**

259 **False** The most frequent features include muscular atrophy and spasticity with exaggeration of tendon reflexes.

260 **False**

PAPER 3 ISQs

Questions

Basic sciences

Basic psychology

1   Instrumental conditioning represents a fundamental procedure under which an association between mental representations of events and actions is formed.

2   Pavlovian conditioning represents a fundamental procedure under which an association between mental representations of events and actions is formed.

3   The learned helplessness model involves exposure to conditions in which responding has no effect on whether reinforcement occurs subsequently.

4   Learned helplessness increases the ability to learn about relationships between responses and reinforcement in general.

5   Learned helplessness results in increased levels of voluntary behaviour.

6   Learned helplessness produces a negative cognitive set.

7   Learned helplessness produces increased levels of aggression.

8   Extinction refers to the decrease in conditioned responses noted if reinforcement is discontinued.

9   Extinction of a conditioned phobic response may be achieved by sustained and repeated exposure to the phobic object.

10 In classical conditioning, informing the subject of the relationship between the conditioned and unconditioned stimulus without actually pairing the two stimuli cannot produce an immediate and apparent conditioned response.

11 A schedule of reinforcement is a procedure that allows a reward to be made contingent upon a response.

12 The term 'vicarious reinforcement' means that observing a response and its outcome strengthen behaviour despite the subject not personally being aware of the outcomes of that behaviour.

13   Flexibility of divided attention is a reliable predictor of a person's likelihood of being in a vehicle accident.

14   Stage models of attention suggest that selectivity can be modelled in terms of a 'bottleneck' in the later stages of processing.

15   The average short-term memory has a digit span of '7 plus or minus 2'.

[answers on page 89]

Behavioural psychology

16   The term 'sick role behaviour' refers to the effect of unconscious denial.

17   The term 'sick role behaviour' is the activity adopted by those who consider themselves to be ill.

18   The term 'sick role behaviour' refers to the measures taken to prevent disease or detect it in the asymptomatic stage.

19   The term 'sick role behaviour' leads to exemption from normal social behaviour.

20   'Sick role behaviour' is particularly prolonged in children compared with adults.

21   Behavioural assessment of an agoraphobic patient includes fear of closed spaces.

22   Behavioural assessment of an agoraphobic patient includes fear of crowds.

23   Behavioural assessment of an agoraphobic patient includes recent life events.

24   Behavioural assessment of an agoraphobic patient includes avoidance of market places.

25   Behavioural assessment of an agoraphobic patient includes family history.

26   Behavioural assessment of phobias includes habituation.

27   Behavioural assessment of phobias includes incubation.

28   Behavioural assessment of phobias includes preparedness.

29   Behavioural assessment of phobias includes assimilation.

30   Behavioural assessment of phobias includes stimulus generalization.

31   Positive reinforcement is a process by which certain consequences of a response enhance the probability that a response will occur.

32   According to learning theory, instrumental learning is a trial and error learning in which a person attempts to solve a problem by trying different actions until one is successful.

[answers on page 89]

Neuropsychology

33   Wechsler's Adult Intelligence Scale–Revised assesses visual–verbal integration.

34   Stroop's Color-Word Interference Test assesses the speed of verbal and non-verbal information.

[answers on page 90]

Human development

35   Jean Piaget is best known for his theories on the importance of infant–mother bonding.

36   According to the classical psychoanalytic theory, obsessive–compulsive personality in an adult is linked to the anal stage of psychosexual development.

37   According to the theories of Erik Erikson, the developmental task of school age (6–11 years) is to resolve the psychosocial crisis of industry versus inferiority.

[answers on page 90]

Psychopharmacology

General principles

38   10 mg of trifluoperazine is equivalent to 100 mg of chlorpromazine.

39   4 mg of droperidol is equivalent to 100 mg of chlorpromazine.

40   2 mg of pimozide is equivalent to 100 mg of chlorpromazine.

41   400 mg of sulpiride is equivalent to 100 mg of chlorpromazine.

42   10 mg of haloperidol is equivalent to 100 mg of chlorpromazine.

[answers on page 90]

Pharmacokinetics

43   First order kinetics means a non-reversible reaction proceeds at an ever-increasing rate as the amount of reacting substance falls.

44   The metabolism of alcohol in human beings follows zero-order kinetics.

45   The concentration of an intravenously administered drug declines in an exponential fashion.

46   The term 'bioavailability' refers to the fraction of drug that has been metabolized.

47   Two dose forms of the same drug with an equal bioavailability are not necessarily bioequivalent.

[answers on page 90]

Pharmacodynamics

48   With reference to neurotransmitters, the major inhibitory transmitters are gamma-aminobutyric acid (GABA) and glycine.

49   With reference to neurotransmitters, the distribution of adrenaline in the brain is mainly in the midbrain and brainstem.

50   With reference to neurotransmitters, glutamate is implicated in learning and memory.

51   According to current scientific knowledge regarding dopamine receptors, D_2 receptors are negatively linked with adenylate cyclase.

52   According to current scientific knowledge regarding dopamine receptors, D_1 receptors are approximately 15 times more sensitive to the action of dopamine than D_2 receptors.

53   According to current scientific knowledge regarding dopamine receptors, D_2 receptors are located presynaptically on the corticostriatal neurones and postsynaptically in the striatum and substantia nigra.

54   According to current scientific knowledge regarding dopamine receptors, D_4 receptor density is highest in basal ganglia.

55   According to current scientific knowledge regarding dopamine receptors, clozapine has a selective affinity for D_5 receptors.

56   With regard to the GABA receptor complex, $GABA_B$ receptors are involved in mediating the effects of barbiturates.

57   With regard to the GABA receptor complex, the effects of GABA are sometimes excitatory.

[answers on page 90]

Adverse drug reactions

58   Haloperidol causes depression of mood in a majority of patients.

59   Alpha-methyldopa causes depression of mood in a majority of patients.

60   Amphetamines cause depression of mood in a majority of patients.

61   Corticosteroids cause depression of mood in a majority of patients.

62   Cimetidine causes depression of mood in a majority of patients.

63   Difficulty in micturition is a common side effect of tricyclic antidepressant drugs.

64   Weight gain is a common side effect of tricyclic antidepressant drugs.

65   Excessive sweating is a common side effect of tricyclic antidepressant drugs.

66   Jaundice is a common side effect of tricyclic antidepressant drugs.

67   Prolongation of P-R interval in the electrocardiogram is common in patients treated with tricyclic antidepressant drugs.

68   A potentially fatal interaction occurs following concomitant administration of a phenelzine and red wine.

69   A potentially fatal interaction occurs following concomitant administration of phenelzine and caffeine.

70   A potentially fatal interaction occurs following concomitant administration of phenelzine and codeine.

71   A potentially fatal interaction occurs following concomitant administration of phenelzine and propranolol.

72   A potentially fatal interaction occurs following concomitant administration of phenelzine and lithium carbonate.

73   Pupillary dilation is a peripheral effect of anticholinergic drugs.

74   Dry mouth is a peripheral effect of anticholinergic drugs.

75   Constriction of bronchi is a peripheral effect of anticholinergic drugs.

76   Increased gastric secretion is a side effect of anticholinergic drugs.

77   Retention of urine is a peripheral effect of anticholinergic drugs.

78   Haloperidol is contraindicated in patients with hepatic failure.

79   Moclobemide is contraindicated in patients with hepatic failure.

80   Dothiepin is contraindicated in patients with hepatic failure.

81   Phenelzine is contraindicated in patients with hepatic failure.

82   Lithium carbonate is contraindicated in patients with hepatic failure.

[answers on page 91]

Psychopathology

Descriptive

83   Changes in intensity are characteristic features of sensory distortions.

84   Tactile hallucinations are a characteristic feature of sensory distortions.

85   Changes in quality are a characteristic feature of sensory distortions.

86   Hyperacusis is a characteristic feature of sensory distortions.

87   Changes in spatial form is a characteristic feature of sensory distortions.

88   Pseudohallucinations are types of mental images.

89   Pseudohallucinations are commonly seen in the state of clouded consciousness.

90   Pseudohallucinations are types of real perceptions.

91   Pseudohallucinations may occur in dreams.

92   Pseudohallucinations are located in the objective space.

93   Denial is a mechanism commonly seen in patients with anorexia nervosa.

94   Denial is a mechanism commonly seen in patients suffering from pathological grief reaction.

95   Denial is a mechanism commonly seen in patients who are depressed.

96   Denial is a mechanism commonly seen in patients suffering from fugue states.

97   Denial is a mechanism commonly seen in patients with bulimia nervosa.

98   Creutzfeldt–Jakob disease is a type of prion dementia.

99   Gerstmann–Sträussler syndrome is a type of prion dementia.

100   Lewy body disease is a type of prion dementia.

101   Kuru is a type of prion dementia.

102   Krabbe's disease is a type of prion dementia.

103   Visual hallucinations are characteristic features of autoscopy.

104   Seeing one's own image is a characteristic feature of autoscopy.

105   Auditory hallucinations are characteristic features of autoscopy.

106   Hysterical behaviour is a characteristic feature of autoscopy.

107   Phantom mirror image phenomenon is a characteristic feature of autoscopy.

108   Hypervigilance is an essential feature of patients with post-traumatic stress disorder.

109   Pervasive anxiety is an essential feature of patients with post-traumatic stress disorder.

110   Anhedonia is an essential feature of patients with post-traumatic stress disorder.

111   Intolerance to alcohol is an essential feature of patients with post-traumatic stress disorder.

112   An exaggerated startle response is an essential feature of patients with post-traumatic stress disorder.

113   Flight of ideas is a characteristic feature of mania.

114   Flight of ideas is a characteristic feature of schizophrenia.

115   Flight of ideas is a characteristic feature of hypothalamic lesions.

116   Flight of ideas is a characteristic feature of schizoaffective disorder.

117   Flight of ideas is a characteristic feature of obsessive–compulsive disorder.

118   Repetition is a characteristic feature of the phenomenon called perseveration.

119   Knight's move is a characteristic feature of the phenomenon called perseveration.

120   Verbal stereotypy is a characteristic feature of the phenomenon called perseveration.

121   Disturbance of the flow of thinking is a characteristic feature of the phenomenon called perseveration.

122   Crowding of thoughts is a characteristic feature of the phenomenon called perseveration.

123   Tactile hallucinations characteristically occur in cocaine psychosis.

124   Tactile hallucinations characteristically occur in Korsakoff's psychosis.

125   Tactile hallucinations characteristically occur in alcoholic hallucinosis.

126   Tactile hallucinations characteristically occur in delirium tremens.

127   Tactile hallucinations characteristically occur in temporal lobe epilepsy.

128   According to the International Classification of Diseases (ICD)-10, the diagnostic criteria of histrionic personality include unwillingness to make even reasonable demands on the people one depends on.

129   According to ICD-10, the diagnostic criteria of histrionic personality include self-dramatization, theatricality and exaggerated expressions of emotion.

130   According to ICD-10, the diagnostic criteria of histrionic personality include suggestibility.

131   According to ICD-10, the diagnostic criteria of histrionic personality include limited capacity to make everyday decisions without an excessive amount of advice and reassurance from others.

132   According to ICD-10, the diagnostic criteria of histrionic personality include over concern with physical attractiveness.

133   Symptoms differentiating major depression from anorexia nervosa include constipation.

134   Symptoms differentiating major depression from anorexia nervosa include loss of weight.

135   Symptoms differentiating major depression from anorexia nervosa include low self-esteem.

136   Symptoms differentiating major depression from anorexia nervosa include early morning waking.

137   Excessive binge eating characteristically occurs in patients with thyrotoxicosis.

138   Excessive binge eating characteristically occurs in patients with anorexia nervosa.

139   Excessive binge eating characteristically occurs in patients with Kleine–Levin syndrome.

140   Excessive binge eating characteristically occurs in patients with social anxiety disorder.

141   Excessive binge eating characteristically occurs in patients suffering from pathological grief reaction.

142   Dissociation characteristically occurs in malingering.

143   Dissociation characteristically occurs in automatic writing.

144   Dissociation characteristically occurs in twilight states.

145   Dissociation characteristically occurs in Ganser's syndrome.

146   Dissociation characteristically occurs in depersonalization–derealization syndrome.

147   The characteristic features which differentiate anorexia nervosa from bulimia nervosa, include body shape disparagement.

148   The characteristic features which differentiate anorexia nervosa from bulimia nervosa, include amenorrhoea.

149   The characteristic features which differentiate anorexia nervosa from bulimia nervosa, include significant weight loss.

150   The characteristic features which differentiate anorexia nervosa from bulimia nervosa, include lanugo hair.

151   The characteristic features which differentiate anorexia nervosa from bulimia nervosa, include selective avoidance of a high-calorie diet.

152   Excessive eating characteristically occurs in patients suffering from normal-weight bulimia.

153   Excessive eating characteristically occurs in patients with Prader–Willi syndrome.

154   Excessive eating characteristically occurs in patients with diabetes mellitus.

155   Excessive eating characteristically occurs in patients with major depression.

156   Excessive eating characteristically occurs in patients suffering from generalized anxiety disorder.

157   The term 'misidentification' refers to a sense of presence of an identical double.

158   Misidentification usually occurs in patients with De Clérambault's syndrome.

159   Misidentification is considered to be a normal experience.

160   Misidentification is a common feature of paranoid schizophrenia.

161   Misidentification is commonly caused by a delusional system.

[answers on page 91]

Dynamic

162   An ego defence mechanism frequently associated with hysterical conversion disorder is identification.

163   An ego defence mechanism frequently associated with hysterical conversion disorder is sublimation.

164   An ego defence mechanism frequently associated with hysterical conversion disorder is projection.

165   An ego defence mechanism frequently associated with hysterical conversion disorder is reaction formation.

166   An ego defence mechanism frequently associated with hysterical conversion disorder is denial.

167   According to traditional Freudian psychoanalytical theory, the manifest content of dreams refers to the material, which the therapist seeks to reveal by means of interpretation.

168   According to traditional Freudian psychoanalytic theory, the features of secondary process thinking are characteristic of the latent content of dreams.

169   According to traditional Freudian psychoanalytic theory, the superego represents the fulfilment of ego ideal.

170   According to traditional Freudian psychoanalytic theory, 'dream work' is the patient's effort to reveal the latent content of dreams.

171   According to traditional Freudian psychoanalytic theory, the 'latency period' causes a resurgence of the sexual drive.

172   Signal anxiety plays an important role in ego defence mechanisms.

173   Actual anxiety plays an important role in ego defence mechanisms.

174   Neurotic anxiety plays an important role in ego defence mechanisms.

175   Panic anxiety plays an important role in ego defence mechanisms.

176   Anxious expectation of harmful retaliatory punishment is called castration anxiety.

177   Anxious expectation of harmful retaliatory punishment is called separation anxiety.

178   Id anxiety often amounts to panic.

179   Id anxiety is frequently seen in early stages of an acute psychotic episode.

180   Id anxiety involves fear that one will lose control of one's impulses.

181   In Freudian psychoanalytic theory, secondary elaboration is part of dream work.

[answers on page 94]

Clinical theory and skills

Aetiology

182   Avoidance conditioning is considered to be involved in the aetiology of nocturnal enuresis.

183   Avoidance conditioning is considered to be involved in the aetiology of social phobia.

184   Avoidance conditioning is considered to be involved in the aetiology of obsessional rituals.

185   Avoidance conditioning is considered to be involved in the aetiology of premature ejaculation.

186   Avoidance conditioning is considered to be involved in the aetiology of exhibitionism.

187   The psychological mechanism of preparedness operates in the aetiology of phobic disorders.

188   The psychological mechanism of covert sensitization operates in the aetiology of phobic disorders.

189   The psychological mechanism of learned helplessness operates in the aetiology of phobic disorders.

190   The psychological mechanism of avoidance learning operates in the aetiology of phobic disorders.

191   The psychological mechanism of repression operates in the aetiology of phobic disorders.

192   There is a history of attempted suicide in about 40 per cent of completed suicides.

193   Completed suicide is most often preceded by an attempted suicide in the previous 3 months.

194   The current trend indicates a shift towards late middle age for the maximum risk of suicide.

195   Patients suffering from antisocial personality disorder are more likely to commit suicide than the general population.

196   Being married offers some protection against suicide.

[answers on page 95]

Diagnosis

197   Past history of concomitant treatment with antidepressant and antipsychotic drugs is strongly suggestive of a diagnosis of schizoaffective disorder.

198   Past history of thought broadcasting is strongly suggestive of a diagnosis of schizoaffective disorder.

199   Past history of intermingling features of schizophrenia and depression is strongly indicative of a diagnosis of schizoaffective disorder.

200   Past history of lithium therapy is strongly suggestive of a diagnosis of schizoaffective disorder.

201   Past history of intermingling features of schizophrenia and mania is strongly indicative of a diagnosis of schizoaffective disorder.

[answers on page 96]

History taking/interviewing

202   Exploration of parapraxes is a psychoanalytic technique.

203   Repression is a psychoanalytic technique.

204   Hypnosis is a psychoanalytic technique.

205   Free association is a psychoanalytic technique.

206   Interpretation of dreams is a psychoanalytic technique.

207 In analytic psychotherapy, the patient is addressed by his or her first name throughout the treatment.

208 In analytic psychotherapy, eye-to-eye contact is necessary for a successful outcome.

209 In analytic psychotherapy, the therapist should direct the patient throughout the treatment.

210 Interpretations of dreams and transference are essential components of analytic psychotherapy.

211 Personality tests can reliably assess premorbid personality.

212 In assessing premorbid personality, one should take into account the patient's personality in the 2 years prior to the index illness.

213 Assessment of premorbid personality should be included in the psychodynamic formulation to increase an understanding of the presenting problem.

214 In assessing premorbid personality, the patient's own appraisal is usually considered adequate.

215 The General Health Questionnaire (GHQ) can reliably assess premorbid personality.

216 In a model psychiatric interview one should start with open-ended questions.

217 As regards a model psychiatric interview, the mental state examination should be performed in a set order.

218 In a model psychiatric interview, occupational and educational history serves as a check on premorbid personality.

219 As regards a model psychiatric interview, family history helps to understand the family dynamics between the family members.

220 Characteristic features of a 'good' interviewer include demeanour of confidence without dogmatism.

221 Characteristic features of a 'good' interviewer include sensitivity to subtleties of verbal human interaction.

222 In a psychiatric interview, engagement is generally facilitated by an initial period of overt attention to the patient's expressed concerns.

223 Routine questions about premorbid personality provide useful information about dissocial personality traits.

[answers on page 96]

Mental state examination

224   Digit span is a standard test of long-term memory.

225   The cognitive estimates test assesses executive functions of the frontal lobes.

226   The serial sevens test serves as an indicator of the mathematical ability of the patient.

227   The serial sevens test is a good indicator of concentration.

228   The serial sevens test is a diagnostic test for Alzheimer's disease.

229   The serial sevens test is able to differentiate cognitive impairment due to a variety of reasons.

230   With regard to the serial sevens test, performance of a psychotic patient is usually impaired.

[answers on page 97]

Classification

231   One of the main features of ICD-10 is that it has been produced in a single but elaborate version.

232   As regards the main features of ICD-10, F30–F39 refer to mood disorders.

233   As regards the main features of ICD-10, the division between neurosis and psychosis is adopted from ICD-9.

234   As regards the main features of ICD-10, the chapter that deals with mental disorders contains 50 categories.

235   As regards the main features of ICD-10, the terms neurosis and psychosis have been excluded throughout the text.

236   According to Diagnostic and Statistics Manual (DSM)-IV, a pattern of unstable and intense interpersonal relationships characterized by alternation between extremes of over-idealization and devaluations is a feature of borderline personality disorder.

237   According to DSM-IV, affective instability is a characteristic feature of borderline personality disorder.

238   According to DSM-IV, reaction to criticism with feelings of rage, shame or humiliation is characteristic feature of borderline personality disorder.

239   According to DSM-IV, preoccupation with feelings of envy is a characteristic feature of borderline personality disorder.

240   According to DSM-IV, chronic feelings of emptiness and boredom are characteristic features of borderline personality disorder.

[answers on page 97]

Physical/neurological examination

241   Presence of akathisia is helpful in the diagnosis of a speech disorder in a 40-year-old man.

242   Presence of pill-rolling tremor is helpful in the diagnosis of a speech disorder in a 40-year-old man.

243   Presence of a mild diastolic murmur at the apex is helpful in the diagnosis of a speech disorder in a 40-year-old man.

244   Presence of nystagmus with intention tremor is helpful in the diagnosis of a speech disorder in a 40-year-old man.

245   Presence of painless indolent ulcers in both hands is helpful in the diagnosis of a speech disorder in a 40-year-old man.

246   Loss of short-term memory is a characteristic feature of frontal lobe dysfunction.

247   Lack of foresight is a characteristic feature of frontal lobe dysfunction.

248   Distractibility is a characteristic feature of frontal lobe dysfunction.

249   Aphasia is a characteristic feature of frontal lobe dysfunction.

250   Depressed mood is a characteristic feature of frontal lobe dysfunction.

251   A brainstem lesion can be clinically distinguished from a cortical lesion by the presence of blurred vision.

252   A brainstem lesion can be clinically distinguished from a cortical lesion by the presence of dysphagia.

253   A brainstem lesion can be clinically distinguished from a cortical lesion by the presence of vertigo.

254   A brainstem lesion can be clinically distinguished from a cortical lesion by the presence of dysphasia.

255   A brainstem lesion can be clinically distinguished from a cortical lesion if paralysis of an upper limb is worse than that of a lower limb.

256   Finger agnosia is a characteristic feature of Gerstmann's syndrome.

257   Dysphasia is a characteristic feature of Gerstmann's syndrome.

258   Right to left orientation is a characteristic feature of Gerstmann's syndrome.

259   Dysgraphia is a characteristic feature of Gerstmann's syndrome.

260   Dyslexia is a characteristic feature of Gerstmann's syndrome.

[answers on page 97]

Answers and explanations

Basic sciences

Basic psychology

1   True
2   True
3   True
4   False
5   False
6   True
7   False
8   True
9   True
10 False
11 True
12 True
13 True
14 True
15 True

Behavioural psychology

16 **False**   Sick role behaviour was first described by Talcott Parsons in 1951. It does not involve any judgement by the doctor regarding whether the processes involved are conscious or unconscious.
17 **True**
18 **False**
19 **True**   The other right of the sick individual is exemption from blame of the illness.
20 **True**   Parsons described two obligations: (i) a wish to recover and (ii) a wish to accept the appropriate help.
21 **True**
22 **True**
23 **False**
24 **True**
25 **False**   Behavioural assessment consists of a highly detailed account of the current determinants of the agoraphobic problem rather than its historical antecedents and predisposing or precipitating factors.
26 **False**   Habituation is based on the theory that the practical idea early in training is repeated and predictably used to elicit thoughts over the period required for anxiety reduction. At the same time, any covert avoidance and neutralizing behaviours are prevented.
27 **False**

28   **True**   The theory of 'preparedness' applies to phobias of small animals, illness, injury, thunderstorms, heights, strangers and water. It also applies to situations such as being far away from a safe place and being rejected by other people. It means that the thing feared may be or have been potentially dangerous to the human race.

29   **False**

30   **True**

31   **True**

32   **True**

Neuropsychology

33   **True**

34   **True**

Human development

35   **False**

36   **True**

37   **True**

Psychopharmacology

General principles

38   **False**   The equivalent dose is 5 mg.

39   **True**

40   **True**

41   **False**   The equivalent dose is 200 mg.

42   **False**   The equivalent dose is 3 mg.

Pharmacokinetics

43   **False**   Most drugs follow first order kinetics. The rate of absorption depends upon the dose remaining to be absorbed. The rate of elimination directly depends on the amount of drug remaining in the body.

44   **True**   It means the rate of absorption is independent of the concentration of the drug.

45   **True**   It follows first order kinetics.

46   **False**   Bioavailability means the fraction of drug that has been absorbed.

47   **True**   Bioequivalence is dependent upon efficacy, which in turn depends on plasma concentration.

Pharmacodynamics

48   **True**

49   **True**

50   **True**   Glycine

51   **True** D_1 receptors are positively linked.

52   **True**

53 **True**
54 **False** It is highest in the frontal cortex and amygdala.
55 **False** D_4 receptors
56 **False** $GABA_A$ mediates the effects of benzodiazepines and barbiturates.
57 **False** They are inhibitory.

Adverse drug reactions

58 **True**
59 **True**
60 **False** They produce euphoria.
61 **True**
62 **False** It is not associated with depression or elevation of mood.
63 **True**
64 **True**
65 **True**
66 **False**
67 **False** The common change in ECG is a prolongation of the QT interval.
68 **True** Alcohol containing tyramine interacts with monoamine oxidase inhibitors (MAOIs) and produces hypertensive crisis.
69 **False** Caffeine is a weak stimulant present in tea and coffee. It is included in many analgesic preparations, but does not contribute to their analgesic or anti-inflammatory effect.
70 **True** MAO inhibitors and opioid–analgesic interactions include CNS excitement or depression, and hypertension or hypotension.
71 **False**
72 **False**
73 **True**
74 **True**
75 **False** Anticholinergic drugs produce relaxation of bronchi.
76 **False** There is reduced gastric secretion.
77 **True**
78 **False**
79 **False** Moclobemide should be avoided in severe hepatic impairment.
80 **False**
81 **True**
82 **False**

Psychopathology

Descriptive

83 **True** In sensory distortions, there is a constant real perceptual object which is perceived in a distorted way, such as changes in intensity, quality and spatial form.
84 **False** It is a type of sensory deception which occurs without an adequate stimulus.

85 **True** See answer 83.

86 **True** The threshold at which sound is perceived as loud is lowered, i.e. there is a generalized increase in sensory input.

87 **True** See answer 83.

88 **True** Although the mental image is clear and vivid, it lacks the substantiality of perceptions.

89 **False** They are seen in full consciousness and are known not to be real perceptions.

90 **False** See answer 89.

91 **False** Dreams occur in rapid eye movement (paradoxical) sleep. Pseudohallucinations are perhaps the most likely phenomenological forms that describe the apocalyptic experience of visions.

92 **False** They are always located in subjective space and perceived with the inner eye or ear.

93 **True**

94 **True**

95 **True**

96 **True**

97 **True** Denial is a direct disavowal of traumatic sensory data. It is ordinarily a defence against the external world of reality when that reality is overwhelmingly disturbing. Although it is associated primarily with psychoses and severe personality disorders, normal people, especially in the face of catastrophic events, may also use it.

98 **True** Prion dementias, i.e. subacute spongiform encephalopathy are characterized by the accumulation in the brain of an abnormal form of a normal host protease-resistant protein, PrP, hence the name 'prion'.

99 **True** It is inherited as an autosomal dominant disorder with complete penetrance.

100 **False** Lewy bodies are eosinophilic intracellular inclusions that are present in the basal ganglia and substantia nigra of patients with Parkinson's disease.

101 **True**

102 **False** It is also known as globoid cell leukodystrophy or galactosyl-ceramide lipidosis, and it is caused by a deficiency of the enzyme galacto-cerebroside-B-galactosidase, which leads to an accumulation of galacto-cerebroside in the central and peripheral nervous systems.

103 **True** It is the experience of seeing oneself and knowing that it is oneself. It may take the form of pseudohallucinations.

104 **True** See answer 103.

105 **False** It may involve several modalities of sensation, but auditory hallucination is not a characteristic feature.

106 **False** Autoscopy is occasionally described as a hysterical behaviour.

107 **True** Phantom mirror image and autoscopy are synonymous.

108 **True**

109 **True**

110 **True**

111 **False**   Excessive use of alcohol or drugs may be a complicating factor.

112 **True**

113 **True**   Flight of ideas is an acceleration of the flow of thinking in which there is no general direction and the connection between successive thoughts appears to be due to chance factors.

114 **False**   It occurs occasionally in excited schizophrenic patients.

115 **True**

116 **True**

117 **False**

118 **True**   In perseveration, a disorder of the continuity of thinking a word, phrase or idea persists beyond the point at which it is relevant.

119 **False**   Knight's move or derailment refers to a transition from one topic to another, either between sentences or in mid-sentence with no logical relation between the two topics.

120 **False**   Here the same word or phrase is used regardless of the situation.

121 **True**

122 **False**   Here the patient describes their thoughts as being passively concentrated and compressed in their head. The associations are experienced as being excessive in amount and outside the patient's control.

123 **True**   Tactile hallucinations, sometimes called haptic hallucinations are experienced as sensations of being touched, pricked or strangled. They may be felt as movements just below the skin which the patient may attribute to insects, worms or other small creatures burrowing through tissues.

124 **False**

125 **False**

126 **True**

127 **False**   Hallucinations of smell, taste, vision, hearing or bodily sensations and distorted perceptions occur in temporal lobe epilepsy.

128 **False**   This is a diagnostic feature of dependent personality disorder.

129 **True**

130 **True**

131 **False**   See answer 128.

132 **True**

133 **False**

134 **False**   Most patients with major depression do not have a desire for excessive weight loss or excessive fear of weight gain, whereas in anorexia nervosa, the weight loss should be at least 15% of normal body weight.

135 **False**   Depressed mood and lability of mood are common features of anorexia nervosa. In chronic cases, hopelessness and thoughts of suicide may be present.

136 **False**

137 **False**   In thyrotoxicosis, there is weight loss in spite of increased appetite.

138 **True**   Up to half of anorexic patients have episodes of uncontrollable overeating, sometimes called bingeing or bulimia.

139 **False**   Klein–Levin syndrome consists of somnolence and increased appetite, often lasting for days or weeks and with long periods of normality between them.

140 **False**

141 **False**

142 **False**   Malingering is the voluntary production and presentation of false or grossly exaggerated physical or psychological symptoms. The symptoms are produced in pursuit of a goal that is obviously recognizable with an understanding of the individual's circumstances rather than of his or her individual psychology.

143 **True**

144 **True**

145 **True**

146 **False**   An awareness of change is present, which is lacking in dissociative disorders.

147 **False**   The body image disturbance is one of the least understood aspects of these disorders. It includes body shape misperception (all or some parts of the body are seen as larger than their actual size) and body shape disparagement (an intense dislike of body or parts of it).

148 **True**

149 **True**

150 **True**

151 **True**   One of the features which distinguishes bulimia nervosa from anorexia nervosa is the profound loss of control over eating.

152 **True**

153 **True**

154 **True**

155 **True**   Most depressed patients complain of loss of appetite. However, some patients eat more and gain weight. It seems that eating brings temporary relief to their distressing feelings.

156 **False**

157 **True**

158 **False**

159 **True**

160 **False**

161 **True**   In schizophrenia, it can be based on a delusional perception. It could also result from an excessive concretization of memory images, so that the person retains all the minute details of the characteristics of the people he or she encounters.

Dynamic

162 **True**   It refers to the unconscious process of taking on some of the activities or characteristics of another person.

163 **False**   In sublimation, the anxieties become channelled into positive acts or ways of life.

164 **False**   It is a means of dealing with uncomfortable emotions or attributes by resisting acknowledging them within oneself and by attributing them to others.

165 **False**   It is characterized by warding off an unacceptable wish or impulse by adopting a character trait that is diametrically opposite to it.

166 **False**   'Conversion' of psychic energy into physical channels and 'repression' are other mental mechanisms involved in dissociative states.

167 **False**   It is the latent or hidden content of the dream that can be interpreted to understand the unconscious issues in the dream.

168 **False**   Secondary process thinking is conscious and based on the reality principle.

169 **False**

170 **True**

171 **False**

172 **True**

173 **False**

174 **False**

175 **False**

176 **True**

177 **False**

178 **True**

179 **True**

180 **True**

181 **True**

Clinical theory and skills

Aetiology

182 **False**

183 **True**

184 **True**   Avoidance of objects or situations, which triggers obsessions, is one of the core features of obsessional problems.

185 **False**

186 **False**   Avoidance or relief from distressing emotion is frequently an immediate effect of problem behaviour. It is often the most potent maintaining factor.

187 **True**   Preparedness is an inherited biological trait and a concept used in learning theory.

188 **False**   It is the use of aversive stimuli in imagination in management of deviant sexual behaviours and urges.

189 **False**   Seligman suggested that depression develops when reward or punishment is no longer clearly contingent upon the action of the organism.

190 **True**

191 **True** The source of anxiety is excluded from consciousness by repression and attached to the manifest object by displacement. A reasonable suggestion is that phobic symptoms are due to a combination of conditioning and abnormal cognition (fear of evaluation).

192 **True**

193 **False**

194 **True**

195 **True**

196 **True**

Diagnosis

197 **False**

198 **True**

199 **True**

200 **True**

201 **True** Schizoaffective disorder is an episodic disorder in which both affective and schizophrenic symptoms are prominent within the same episode of illness, preferably simultaneously, but at least within a few days of each other. Such patients usually respond to electroconvulsive therapy, antipsychotics and antimanic drugs, but often not to tricyclic antidepressant drugs.

History taking/interviewing

202 **True**

203 **False** It is an ego defence mechanism, which operates unconsciously by expelling unacceptable wishes and feelings or fantasies from conscious awareness.

204 **False**

205 **True**

206 **True**

207 **False** It is good practice to call the patient by his or her first name, but only with the patient's permission.

208 **False**

209 **False** The therapist must simply create an atmosphere in which the patient feels free to talk. The therapist can learn a great deal by allowing the patient to ramble freely for a while.

210 **False** Interpretations are made about the patient's behaviour within or outside the therapeutic sessions. These include acting out, counter transference, parapraxes, unconscious conflict, deficits and distortions of intrapsychic structures.

211 **False** Aspects of a person's premorbid personality can be judged by asking him or her for their self-rating, by asking other people who know them well, and by observing their behaviour at the interview.

212 **False** Good indicators of premorbid personality can often be obtained by asking the patient or others how he or she has behaved in particular circumstances.

213 **True**

214 **True**   The patient's own account of his or her personality may be distorted by their illness or a general lack of insight.

215 **False**   The GHQ is a self-rated, 60-item questionnaire designed to identify psychiatric 'cases'. It was designed for use in a community setting, primary care or general medical outpatient setting.

216 **True**

217 **True**

218 **True**

219 **True**   The psychiatric interview serves as a psychiatrist's main tool of investigation. It is a technique of obtaining information and serves as a standard situation in which the patient's emotions and attitudes are assessed.

220 **True**

221 **True**

222 **True**

223 **False**

Mental state examination

224 **False**

225 **True**

226 **False**

227 **True**

228 **False**   Performance is grossly impaired in Alzheimer's disease, but the test is not diagnostic.

229 **False**   Performance depends on educational and intellectual attainment and arithmetic skills.

230 **False**   Performance *may* be impaired in psychotic patients.

Classification

231 **False**   ICD-10 is available in several different versions.

232 **True**

233 **False**   The terms 'neurosis' and 'psychosis' are not adopted; however, words such as 'neurotic' and 'psychotic' are used in descriptive terms.

234 **False**   The chapter that deals with mental disorders has 100 categories.

235 **False**

236 **True**

237 **True**

238 **False**   It is a diagnostic feature of narcissistic personality disorder.

239 **False**

240 **True**

Physical/neurological examination

241 **True**

242 **True** The patient with postencephalitic Parkinson's disease speaks slowly and articulates poorly, slurring over many syllables and trailing off at the end of sentences. The voice is low-pitched, monotonous and lacks inflection.

243 **False**

244 **True** In cerebellar lesions, the principal speech abnormality is slowness, imprecise enunciation, monotony and unnatural separation of syllables.

245 **True** Syringobulbia, which never occurs without syringomyelia, may extend into the lateral tegmentum of the medulla. There is unilateral paralysis of the palate and vocal cords, as well as weakness and atrophy of one side of the tongue.

246 **True**

247 **True** It is a failure to anticipate the consequence of a course of action.

248 **True**

249 **False**

250 **False**

251 **False** The causes of blurred vision vary with age and include myopia, presbyopia, cataracts, glaucoma, retinal haemorrhages and detachments.

252 **True**

253 **True** Vertigo of brain stem origin implicates vestibular nuclei and their connections. In these cases, auditory function is nearly always spared. There are attendant signs of involvement of cranial nerves, sensory and motor tracts and nystagmus.

254 **False** Dysphasia may also occur in cortical lesions.

255 **False**

256 **True** Gerstmann's syndrome is a particular form of body image disturbance resulting from a dominant parietal lobe lesion. Other features include acalculia and colour agnosia. The condition may occur in the absence of any other form of body image disturbance.

257 **False**

258 **False**

259 **True**

260 **False**

PAPER 4 ISQs

Questions

Basic sciences

Basic psychology

1   Cognitive dissonance paradoxically produces a state of comfort and relaxation.

2   The term 'cognitive dissonance' refers to the disharmony between a person's beliefs, knowledge and behaviour.

3   A response is less likely to be extinguished if it was established during partial reinforcement.

4   In self-serving bias, one's own failures are attributed to situational factors.

5   Rorschach's test is an objective test of personality.

6   The term 'synaesthesia' refers to the ability to associate images in one sensory modality (such as vision) with another sensory modality (such as sound).

7   Memory is sensitive to the circumstances of both learning and retrieval and is particularly impaired when these are incompatible.

8   Classical conditioning is an example of associative learning.

9   Operant conditioning is an example of associative learning.

10   Acquisition stage of conditioning is the period during which an association is being acquired between the conditioned stimulus and the unconditioned stimulus.

11   According to Thornidike's law of effect, a voluntary behaviour that is paired with subsequent reward is weakened.

12   According to learning theory, a negative reinforcer is an aversive stimulus whose removal increases the probability of occurrence of the operant behaviour.

13   According to learning theory, punishment is a situation that occurs if an aversive stimulus is presented whenever a given behaviour occurs.

14   According to learning theory, the need for food and water is an example of a primary reinforcer.

15   According to learning theory, the need for money is an example of a secondary reinforcer.

16   The term 'halo effect' refers to a source of error in which the observer allows his or her preconception based on a feature of general attitude to influence the responses so that they tend to fit in with this preconception.

17   The term 'Hawthorne effect' refers to the influence of the social interactions of the subject with the observer on the responses.

18   'Arbitrary abstraction' is considered to be a negative automatic thought in depressed patients.

19   'Overgeneralization' is considered to be a negative automatic thought in depressed patients.

20   'Selective abstraction' is considered to be a negative automatic thought in depressed patients.

21   'Dichotomous reasoning' is considered to be a negative automatic thought in depressed patients.

22   'Categorization' is considered to be a negative automatic thought in depressed patients.

[answers on page 113]

Behavioural psychology

23   According to behavioural psychology, imprinting is implicated in the pathogenesis of specific phobias.

24   According to behavioural psychology, learned helplessness is implicated in the pathogenesis of specific phobias.

25   According to behavioural psychology, preparedness is implicated in the pathogenesis of specific phobias.

26   According to behavioural psychology, incubation is implicated in the pathogenesis of specific phobias.

27   According to behavioural psychology, the second order conditioning is implicated in the pathogenesis of specific phobias.

28   In primary reward conditioning, the learnt response is instrumental in obtaining a non-biologically significant reward.

29   In secondary reward learning, the learnt response is instrumental in obtaining a biologically significant reward.

30   According to learning theory, primary reinforcers are completely independent of a previous learning process.

31   According to learning theory, secondary reinforcers are based on previously rewarded learning process.

32   According to learning theory, negative reinforcement is related to escape learning.

[answers on page 113]

Neuropsychology

33   Benton's Verbal Fluency Test assesses the speed of verbal information processing.

34   The Halstead–Reitan Neurological Battery includes normative data for psychiatric population.

35   Memory is significantly impaired in frontal lobe lesions.

36   Non-dominant temporal lobe lesions lead to an impairment of the ability to reproduce a picture from memory.

37   The Wisconsin Card Sorting Test is a specific test for detecting impairment of frontal lobe functions.

38   Dementia of frontal lobe type results in early impairment of verbal fluency.

[answers on page 114]

Human development

39   The psychoanalyst Erik Erikson hypothesized that the development of the human ego proceeds through eight identifiable stages from birth onwards, marked by specific psychosocial crises.

40   Normal parent–infant behaviour is best described in interaction terms as an example of complementary affiliative behaviour.

41   Masturbation and sexual play with other children in early childhood are generally regarded as normal behaviour at this stage of development.

[answers on page 114]

Pharmacology

General principles

42   Citalopram is an example of a selective serotonin reuptake inhibitor drug.

43   Buspirone is an example of a selective serotonin reuptake inhibitor drug.

44   Zopiclone is an example of a selective serotonin reuptake inhibitor drug.

45   Maprotiline is an example of a selective serotonin reuptake inhibitor drug.

46   Moclobemide is an example of reversible monoamine oxidase (MAO) type B antidepressant drugs.

[answers on page 114]

Pharmacokinetics

47   All orally administered antipsychotic drugs are subject to presystemic extraction with passage through the liver.

48   The extent of first pass effects of antipsychotic drugs depends on their clearance, which is capacity limited.

49   As regards the pharmacokinetics of antipsychotic depot preparations, their bioavailability is limited by the rate of metabolism.

50   First bypass metabolism enhances the passage of psychotropic drugs through the blood–brain barrier.

51   With reference to the pharmacokinetics of chlorpromazine, its plasma level increases with concomitant administration of a tricyclic antidepressant drug.

52   With reference to the pharmacokinetics of chlorpromazine, its plasma concentration decreases with concomitant administration of a selective serotonin reuptake inhibitor drug.

53   With reference to the pharmacokinetics of chlorpromazine, a peak plasma concentration is achieved approximately 3 hours after an oral dose.

54   With reference to the pharmacokinetics of chlorpromazine, its therapeutic effect is directly proportional to the plasma concentration of drug.

55   With reference to the pharmacokinetics of chlorpromazine, its plasma concentration decreases with concomitant administration of an anticholinergic drug.

[answers on page 114]

Pharmacodynamics

56   The efficacy of the new generation of antipsychotic drugs relies on the combination of D_2 antagonism and a powerful degree of 5-HT_{2A} antagonism.

57   Phenelzine has an approximately 6:1 preference for type A MAO enzyme.

58   Moclobemide is a selective inhibitor of type B MAO enzyme.

59   The clinical effects of lithium depend on its action on second messenger systems.

60   Benzodiazepines facilitate the inhibitory effects of gamma-aminobutyric acid (GABA) on the central nervous system by prolonging the duration of opening of chloride channels.

61   With regard to the GABA receptor complex, chloride channels open when GABA binds to a postsynaptic GABA.

62   GABA binds to benzodiazepine receptors.

63   With regard to receptor ligands, an agonist has its characteristic effect at the receptor of the 'normal' transmitter substance.

64   With regard to receptor ligands, anticonvulsant drugs are 'inverse' agonists at benzodiazepine receptors.

65   With regard to receptor ligands, an agonist at the benzodiazepine receptors appears to enhance the binding of GABA to its receptors.

66   High molecular weight enhances the passage of psychotropic drugs through the blood–brain barrier.

[answers on page 114]

Adverse drug reactions

67   Phenelzine produces a sedative effect in therapeutic doses.

68   Dothiepin produces a sedative effect in therapeutic doses.

69   Trazodone produces a sedative effect in therapeutic doses.

70   Fluoxetine produces a sedative effect in therapeutic doses.

71   Fluvoxamine produces a sedative effect in the majority of patients in therapeutic doses.

72   Moclobemide produces a sedative effect in the majority of patients in therapeutic doses.

73   Haloperidol produces a sedative effect in the majority of patients in therapeutic doses.

74   Risperidone produces a sedative effect in the majority of patients in therapeutic doses.

75   Nortriptyline produces a sedative effect in the majority of patients in therapeutic doses.

76   Sertraline produces a sedative effect in the majority of patients in therapeutic doses.

[answers on page 115]

Psychopathology

Descriptive

77 Confabulation is a characteristic feature of Korsakoff's psychosis.

78 Confabulation is almost always associated with clouding of consciousness.

79 Confabulation is due to a disorder of temporal sequence of events.

80 Confabulation is proportional to the degree of anterograde amnesia.

81 Confabulation is frequently seen in patients with chronic schizophrenia.

82 Diplopia is a characteristic feature of generalized anxiety disorder.

83 An intention tremor is a characteristic feature of generalized anxiety disorder.

84 Frequent yawning is a characteristic feature of generalized anxiety disorder.

85 Digital paraesthesia is a characteristic feature of generalized anxiety disorder.

86 Subjective difficulty in breathing is a characteristic feature of generalized anxiety disorder.

87 The characteristic features that differentiate depression from anorexia nervosa include cold peripheries.

88 The characteristic features that differentiate depression from anorexia nervosa include bradycardia.

89 The characteristic features that differentiate depression from anorexia nervosa include overactivity.

90 The characteristic features that differentiate depression from anorexia nervosa include psychomotor retardation.

91 The characteristic features that differentiate depression from anorexia nervosa include poor appetite.

92 Early morning waking is a typical feature of depression.

93 Anhedonia is a typical feature of depression.

94 Increased fatigability is a typical feature of depression.

95 Diurnal variation in mood is a typical feature of depression.

96 Increased libido is a typical feature of depression.

97 Depression may be a presenting symptom of gastric carcinoma.

98 Depression may be a presenting symptom of hypothyroidism.

99 Depression may be a presenting symptom of phaeochromocytoma.

100 Depression may be a presenting symptom of Alzheimer's disease.

101 Depression may be a presenting symptom of pancreatic carcinoma.

102 Anxiety is a recognized feature of vitamin B_{12} deficiency.

103 Depression is a recognized feature of vitamin B_{12} deficiency.

104 Paranoid states are a recognized feature of vitamin B_{12} deficiency.

105 Delirium is a recognized feature of vitamin B_{12} deficiency.

106 Short-term impairment of memory is a recognized feature of vitamin B_{12} deficiency.

107 In late paraphrenia genetic predisposition is considered insignificant.

108 With regard to late paraphrenia, the incidence rate is equal in both sexes.

109 Patients with late paraphrenia usually have a previous history of schizophrenia.

110 Sensory deprivation may be an important factor in the aetiology of late paraphrenia.

111 Late paraphrenia is considered to be an early manifestation of Alzheimer's disease.

112 Schneider's first rank symptoms are pathognomonic features of schizophrenia.

113 Schneider's first rank symptoms are present in patients with schizophrenia around the world.

114 Schneider's first rank symptoms are not usually found in psychotic patients with learning disability.

115 Schneider's first rank symptoms are typical of psychotic disorders associated with temporal lobe epilepsy.

116 Schneider's first rank symptoms include Gedankenlautwerden.

117 Inappropriate affect is a negative symptom of schizophrenia.

118 Blunted affect is a negative symptom of schizophrenia.

119 Apathy is a negative symptom of schizophrenia.

120 Indifference to the environment is a negative symptom of schizophrenia.

121 Poverty of movement is a negative symptom of schizophrenia.

122 Loss of pubic hair is a characteristic feature of anorexia nervosa.

123 Loss of at least 25 per cent of body weight is a characteristic feature of anorexia nervosa.

124   Amenorrhoea before significant weight loss is a characteristic feature of anorexia nervosa.

125   Presence of lanugo hair is a characteristic feature of anorexia nervosa.

126   Loss of libido is a characteristic feature of anorexia nervosa.

127   Convulsions are a recognized feature of narcolepsy.

128   Sudden loss of muscle tone is a recognized feature of narcolepsy.

129   Abnormal findings on electroencephalography (EEG) is a recognized feature of narcolepsy.

130   Visual hallucinations are recognized features of narcolepsy.

131   Night terrors are a recognized feature of narcolepsy.

132   Pseudohallucinations are a recognized feature of borderline personality disorder.

133   Pseudohallucinations are a recognized feature of hypnagogic states.

134   Pseudohallucinations are a recognized feature of bereavement.

135   Pseudohallucinations are a recognized feature of chronic fatigue syndrome.

136   Pseudohallucinations are a recognized feature of hypnopompic states.

137   Carl Schneider first described thought echo.

138   Carl Schneider first described 'Made' experiences.

139   Derailment was first described by Carl Schneider

140   Carl Schneider first described substitution.

141   Carl Schneider first described thought broadcasting.

142   When a patient says, 'I heard a voice telling me I was going to be killed', it is an example of Schneider's first rank symptom.

143   When a patient says, 'I know the woman next to me could hear what I was thinking', it is an example of Schneider's first rank symptom.

144   When a patient says, 'I saw the postman dropping a letter and I knew there was going to be nuclear war', it is an example of Schneider's first rank symptom.

145   When a patient says, 'It was a strange force inside my brain that made me break the door', it is an example of Schneider's first rank symptom.

146   When a patient says, 'I don't seem to be able to think for myself. All my thoughts seem to be my father's', it is an example of Schneider's first rank symptom.

147   As regards the assessment of suicidal risk, suicidal intent can vary in severity over a short period of time.

148   As regards the assessment of suicidal risk, asking questions about suicidal ideation increases the actual risk.

149   As regards the assessment of suicidal risk, denial of intent implies a relatively high risk.

150   As regards the assessment of suicidal risk, an admission of the suicide intent minimizes the eventual risk.

151   As regards the assessment of suicidal risk, a previous history of a deliberate self-harm indicates a relatively high risk.

152   Obsessional thoughts are intrusive and disturbing for the patient.

153   Obsessional thoughts are rarely pleasurable.

154   Obsessional thoughts also occur in healthy people.

155   Obsessional thoughts rarely include images.

156   With reference to obsessional thoughts the patient usually acts upon them.

157   The clinical features differentiating pain of psychological origin from pain of physical origin include an increase in severity with passage of time.

158   The clinical features differentiating pain of psychological origin from pain of physical origin include an intermittent course.

159   The clinical features differentiating pain of psychological origin from pain of physical origin include a precise anatomical location.

160   The clinical features differentiating pain of psychological origin from pain of physical origin include relief by placebo.

161   The clinical features differentiating pain of psychological origin from pain of physical origin include relief by analgesics.

162   Emotional lability is a characteristic feature of delirium tremens.

163   Emotional lability is a characteristic feature of bipolar affective disorder.

164   Emotional lability is a characteristic feature of histrionic personality.

165   Emotional lability is a characteristic feature of Alzheimer's disease.

166   Emotional lability is a characteristic feature of simple schizophrenia.

[answers on page 115]

Dynamic psychopathology

167 Denial characteristically occurs in patients with bipolar affective disorder.

168 Denial characteristically occurs in patients with dissocial personality disorder.

169 Denial characteristically occurs in patients suffering from dissociative states.

170 Denial characteristically occurs in patients suffering from a terminal illness.

171 Denial characteristically occurs in patients suffering from anorexia nervosa.

172 According to Freud's psychoanalytic theory, the ego is entirely conscious.

173 According to Freud's psychoanalytic theory, the id is entirely unconscious.

174 According to Freud's psychoanalytic theory, the ego operates on secondary process thinking.

175 According to Freud's psychoanalytic theory, instinct is inherited and unchangeable.

176 According to Freud's psychoanalytic theory, the superego is derived from the ego.

177 The concept of archetypes is associated with Carl Jung.

178 The concept of dream work is associated with Carl Jung.

179 The concept of animus is associated with Carl Jung.

180 The concept of inferiority complex is associated with Carl Jung.

181 The concept of transitional object is associated with Carl Jung.

182 The concept of free association is connected with Carl Jung.

183 The concept of persona is associated with Carl Jung.

184 The concept of anima is associated with Carl Jung.

185 The concept of depressive position is associated with Carl Jung.

186 The concept of character armour is associated with Carl Jung.

187 In psychoanalytic terms, anxiety diminishes in old age.

188 In psychoanalytic terms, anxiety leads to repression.

189 In psychoanalytic terms, anxiety can be a threat to the superego.

190   In psychoanalytic terms, anxiety can be a warning to the ego.

191   In psychoanalytic terms, anxiety is due to unresolved psychic conflicts.

[answers on page 118]

Clinical theory and skills

Aetiology

192   According to the psychoanalytic theory of anxiety, birth trauma is an important factor in its aetiology.

193   According to the psychoanalytic theory of anxiety, bereavement is an important factor in its aetiology.

194   According to the psychoanalytic theory of anxiety, fear of castration is an important factor in its aetiology.

195   According to the psychoanalytic theory of anxiety, separation in childhood is an important factor in its aetiology.

196   According to the psychoanalytic theory of anxiety, maternal deprivation is an important factor in its aetiology.

197   Learning theories have made a significant contribution to the aetiological understanding of agoraphobia.

198   Learning theories have made a significant contribution to the aetiological understanding of social phobia.

199   Learning theories have made a significant contribution to the aetiological understanding of obsessive–compulsive disorder.

200   Learning theories have made a significant contribution to the aetiological understanding of fetishism.

201   Learning theories have made a significant contribution to the aetiological understanding of dissociative states.

202   Inadequate information is one of the factors that influence the occurrence of sexual dysfunction.

203   Poor sex education is one of the factors that influence the occurrence of sexual dysfunction.

204   Depression is one of the factors that influence the occurrence of sexual dysfunction.

205   Loss of attraction is one of the factors that influence the occurrence of sexual dysfunction.

[answers on page 119]

Diagnosis/classification

206 Attention deficit hyperactivity disorder is an axis I diagnosis in the Diagnostic and Statistical Manual (DSM)-IV.

207 Mild mental retardation is an axis I diagnosis in the DSM-IV.

208 Schizotypal disorder is an axis I diagnosis in the DSM-IV.

209 Borderline personality disorder is an axis I diagnosis in the DSM-IV.

210 Late paraphrenia is an axis I diagnosis in the DSM-IV.

211 According to the International Classification of Diseases (ICD)-10, dissociative states include somatoform disorders.

212 According to ICD-10, dissociative states include Ganser's syndrome.

213 According to ICD-10, dissociative states include neurasthenia.

214 According to ICD-10, dissociative states include multiple personality disorder.

215 According to ICD-10, dissociative states include hypochondriasis.

216 Reliability of psychiatric diagnosis is improved by operational definitions.

217 Reliability of psychiatric diagnosis is improved by multiaxial classification.

218 Reliability of psychiatric diagnosis does not matter if the diagnostic categories have low validity.

219 Reliability of psychiatric diagnosis is improved by semistructured interviews.

220 Reliability of psychiatric diagnosis is not significantly different between unstructured and structured interviews.

[answers on page 120]

History taking/interviewing

221 'What can I do for you?' is an open-ended question in a psychiatric interview.

222 'Well, it seems that you are in trouble' is an open-ended question in a psychiatric interview.

223 'Tell me what is troubling you' is an open-ended question in a psychiatric interview.

224 'How are you feeling at the moment?' is an open-ended question in a psychiatric interview.

225 'So, are you less depressed now?' is an open-ended question in a psychiatric interview.

226 In a typical psychiatric interview, as a first step the interviewer should give the patient a pro forma to fill in as soon as he or she arrives.

227 In a typical psychiatric interview, as a first step the interviewer should ask the patient to give the history in his or her own words.

228 In a typical psychiatric interview, as a first step the interviewer should ask the patient about his or her main problem.

229 In a typical psychiatric interview, as a first step the interviewer should make the patient lie on the couch.

230 In a typical psychiatric interview, as a first step the patient should undergo a cursory physical examination by the interviewer.

231 A failure to ask about a history of alcohol abuse is considered to be a pitfall in correctly assessing the patient's mood.

232 A failure to ask direct questions is considered to be a pitfall in correctly assessing the patient's mood.

233 A failure to utilize standardized rating scales is considered to be a pitfall in correctly assessing the patient's mood.

234 An inability to recognize the interviewer's own non-verbal behaviour is considered to be a pitfall in correctly assessing the patient's mood.

235 A failure to interact with the patient's non-verbal communication is considered to be a pitfall in correctly assessing the patient's mood.

236 Special skill is required in conducting a psychiatric interview because the patients usually do not give correct information.

237 Special skill is required in conducting a psychiatric interview because the patient is embarrassed about their symptoms.

238 Special skill is required in conducting a psychiatric interview because the patients usually cannot remember the necessary details.

239 Special skill is required in conducting a psychiatric interview because the patients may be afraid of legal consequences of their answers.

240 Special skill is required in conducting a psychiatric interview because some patients are too psychotic to offer accurate information.

[answers on page 121]

Mental state examination

241 The first clinical examination of a patient with a suspected mental disorder should include a mental state examination.

242 Clinical assessment of a patient with a mental disorder should include a physical examination.

243   Clinical assessment of a patient with a mental disorder should include laboratory studies.

244   Clinical assessment of a patient with a mental disorder is not complete without psychological tests.

245   Clinical assessment of a patient with mental disorder should include screening for organic illness.

246   The psychiatric interview should always be conducted in a quiet office.

247   The psychiatric interview should usually be conducted in the presence of family members.

248   The psychiatric interview should always be conducted with complete confidentiality.

249   The psychiatric interview should always be conducted at eye level with the patient.

250   If a patient believes that Scotland Yard is listening to her telephone conversation, the physician should explain to the patient what a delusion is.

[answers on page 121]

Physical/neurological examination

251   Inability to learn new routes is a characteristic deficit associated with lesions of the non-dominant temporal lobe.

252   Diminution in musical appreciative capacity is a characteristic deficit associated with lesions of the non-dominant temporal lobe.

253   Difficulty in reproducing visual designs from memory is a characteristic deficit associated with lesions of the non-dominant temporal lobe.

254   Persistent emotional instability is a characteristic feature associated with lesions of the non-dominant temporal lobe.

255   Persistent aggressive behaviour is a characteristic feature associated with lesions of the non-dominant temporal lobe.

256   Nystagmus is a characteristic feature of Wernicke's encephalopathy.

257   Ataxia of gait is a characteristic feature of Wernicke's encephalopathy.

258   Tremors of the lips are characteristic feature of Wernicke's encephalopathy.

259   Peripheral neuropathy is a characteristic feature of Wernicke's encephalopathy.

260   Pernicious anaemia is characteristically associated with Wernicke's encephalopathy.

[answers on page 122]

Answers and explanations

Basic sciences

Basic psychology

1 False
2 True
3 True
4 True
5 False
6 True
7 True
8 True
9 True
10 True
11 False
12 True
13 True
14 True
15 True
16 True
17 True
18 False The correct term is 'arbitrary inference', which includes making conclusions on the basis of inadequate information.
19 False In 'overgeneralization', the person is likely to make sweeping judgements based on single instances.
20 False In 'selective abstraction', attention is paid only to the negative aspects of an experience.
21 True In 'dichotomous reasoning', the person tends to think in terms of extremes.
22 False

Behavioural psychology

23 False Imprinting, an ethological concept leads to attachment behaviour learned during a critical period of life.
24 False Learned helplessness implicates that one has no control over the environment. Reduced voluntary movement occurs in depression.
25 True
26 True
27 False
28 False It is instrumental in obtaining a biologically significant reward.
29 False It is instrumental in obtaining non-biologically significant reward.
30 True

31 **True**
32 **True**

Neuropsychology

33 **False** It assesses fluency and word-finding ability. The person is required to say as many words as he or she can, beginning with specific letters of the alphabet in 1 minute.
34 **True**
35 **False**
36 **True**
37 **True**
38 **True**

Human development

39 **True**
40 **True**
41 **True**

Pharmacology

General principles

42 **True**
43 **False** It is an azaspirodecanedione-type anxiolytic drug.
44 **False** It is a cyclopyrolone hypnotic drug.
45 **False** It is a selective noradrenaline reuptake inhibitor antidepressant drug.
46 **False** It is a reversible monoamine oxidase type A inhibitor antidepressant drug.

Pharmacokinetics

47 **True**
48 **False** It is flow limited and not capacity limited.
49 **False** The bioavailability is limited by the rate of absorption of the drug.
50 **False**
51 **True** Chlorpromazine inhibits hepatic enzymes, which may result in reduced metabolism of tricyclic antidepressant drugs leading to higher plasma levels and enhanced effects.
52 **False**
53 **True**
54 **True**
55 **True** Anticholinergic drugs slow gastric emptying leading to delay in their systemic absorption.

Pharmacodynamics

56 **True**
57 **True**

58   **False**   It is a selective inhibitor of type A MAO enzyme.
59   **True**   There are three main neurochemical levels: membrane neurophysiology, neurotransmitters and second messenger systems.
60   **False**   By increasing the number of channels opened.
61   **True**
62   **False**
63   **True**
64   **False**   They are convulsant and anxiogenic. Inverse agonists have the action opposite to agonists.
65   **True**
66   **True**

Adverse drug reactions

67   **False**   Drowsiness but not sedation is one of the common side effects of phenelzine.
68   **True**   Sedation is one of the commonest side effects due to the noradrenergic and histaminergic actions of the drug.
69   **True**   See answer 68.
70   **False**   Drowsiness but not sedation is a common side effect.
71   **False**   See answer 70.
72   **False**
73   **False**   Drowsiness but not sedation is one of the commonest side effects.
74   **False**   See answer 73.
75   **False**   Drowsiness but not sedation is a common side effect in therapeutic doses.
76   **False**

Psychopathology

Descriptive

77   **True**
78   **False**
79   **True**
80   **False**
81   **False**   In schizophrenia there is falsification of memory with persecutory content, but this is not considered to be a frequent feature.
82   **False**
83   **False**   It is a feature of cerebellar disorders.
84   **False**
85   **True**
86   **True**   The characteristic features of generalized anxiety disorder are broadly grouped into four categories: muscle tension, autonomic hyperactivity, apprehensive expectation and problems with vigilance and scanning.
87   **False**

88 True
89 False
90 True   Anorexic patients are usually alert, even though they are emaciated.
91 True   Except in longstanding cases, appetite for food persists and for this reason, the term 'anorexia' is a misnomer.
92 True
93 True
94 True
95 False
96 False   To make a diagnosis of depression, there should be presence of depressed mood, anhedonia, or increased fatigability or all three. In addition, other symptoms (such as reduced self-esteem and self-confidence, ideas of guilt and unworthiness, reduced appetite) are necessary.
97 True
98 True
99 True   Phaeochromocytomas are rare and easily overlooked because of episodic attacks of anxiety. However, depression may be a presenting symptom.
100 True   Presentation of Alzheimer's disease is often with minor forgetfulness, which is difficult to distinguish from ageing. The mood may be predominantly depressed, euphoric, flattened or labile.
101 True
102 False
103 True
104 True
105 True
106 True   The mental symptoms may accompany pernicious anaemia and sub-acute combined degeneration of the spinal cord or precede them by many months.
107 True
108 False
109 False
110 True
111 False
112 False   The term 'late paraphrenia' is some times used as an omnibus term to describe paranoid illnesses presenting for the first time in middle or late age. A high proportion of these patients are single, divorced or widowed with a female preponderance. Deafness is common.
113 True
114 False
115 False
116 True   Gedankenlautwerden means audible thoughts ('echo de la pensée' in French), i.e. the patient hears his or her own thoughts said out loud.
117 True
118 True
119 True

120 **True**

121 **False**   Frank Fish and Hughlings Jackson in the nineteenth century tried to distinguish between positive and negative symptoms on the basis of reduction or loss of normal cerebral function. Poverty of speech and blunted affect are the other negative symptoms of schizophrenia.

122 **False**   Axillary and pubic hair are preserved and there is no breast atrophy.

123 **False**   Body weight is maintained at least 15 per cent below that expected (Quetelet's body mass index is 17.5 or less).

124 **True**   In about a fifth of cases, amenorrhoea precedes weight loss.

125 **True**   Fine downy lanugo hair is sometimes found on the back, arms and sides of the face.

126 **True**   It is the male equivalent of amenorrhoea (Quetelet's body mass index = weight in kg/height in m^2).

127 **False**

128 **False**   Cataplexy, a sudden loss of muscle tone is one of the main features of polysymptomatic narcolepsy.

129 **False**   The electroencephalogram (EEG) shows normal findings with abnormally rapid onset of rapid eye movement sleep during an afternoon nap or the abnormally rapid onset of stage 1 sleep during a multiple daytime EEG sleep.

130 **True**

131 **False**   In night terror, the child wakes up with intense anxiety or terror, accompanied by complete amnesia for the experience on waking.

132 **False**   In borderline personality disorder, there is a pervasive pattern of instability of interpersonal relationships, self-image and affects. There is a marked impulsivity.

133 **False**

134 **True**   Pseudohallucinations are abnormal phenomena that do not meet the criteria for hallucinations. They are figurative and are located in subjective space and perceived with the inner eye or ear.

135 **False**   True hallucinations may occur in healthy people, especially when tired.

136 **False**   Hypnagogic and hypnopompic hallucinations may be visual, auditory or tactile. They occur while falling asleep and during awakening, respectively.

137 **False**

138 **False**

139 **False**

140 **False**

141 **False**   The items in questions 137–141 were described by Kurt Schneider. However, Carl Schneider described five features of formal thought disorder: derailment, substitution, omission, fusion and drivelling.

142 **False**   This is an example of second person auditory hallucination, which does not point to a particular diagnosis. However, its content and especially the patient's reaction may do so.

143 **True** It is an example of thought broadcasting.
144 **True** It is an example of delusional perception.
145 **True** Is is an example of passivity feeling.
146 **True** It is an example of thought insertion.
147 **True**
148 **False** Asking direct questions about suicidal ideation or intent may in fact reduce the risk, as the patient may feel relieved.
149 **False**
150 **False** Denial of suicide intent does not necessarily imply a high risk. The most obvious warning sign is a direct statement of intent. About two-thirds of those who die by suicide have told someone of their intention.
151 **True**
152 **True**
153 **True**
154 **True**
155 **False**
156 **False** Obsessions are recurrent, persistent thoughts, impulses, or images that enter the mind despite the person's efforts to exclude them. The person often regards them as his or her own, and untrue or senseless. The person finds them distressing or unpleasant.
157 **True**
158 **False**
159 **True**
160 **False**
161 **False**
162 **True**
163 **True**
164 **True**
165 **True**
166 **False** The patient may exhibit a blunted or flattened affect. When emotions change in an excessively rapid and abrupt way, the affect is said to be labile.

Dynamic psychopathology

167 **False**
168 **True**
169 **True**
170 **True**
171 **True** Denial is a form of defence against anxiety and it refers to the inability of the individual to acknowledge some reality.
172 **False** The conscious aspect of the ego is the executive organ of the psyche, responsible for decision making and integrating perceptual data. The unconscious aspect of the ego contains defence mechanisms, which are necessary to counteract the powerful instinctual drives harboured in the id.

173 **True** It is only interested in discharging tension. Both the unconscious aspects of the ego and the superego control it.

174 **True** Secondary process thinking is logical, rational and geared to meet the demands of real life.

175 **True** It represents all the inherited biological and constitutional features of basic drives such as aggression, sex, eating and elimination.

176 **False** The superego is built up from internalized representations of the standards and ideals upheld by others who are particularly important to us.

177 **True** Archetypes are generalized symbols and images within the collective unconscious, which refers to the myths common to all mankind.

178 **False** It is associated with Sigmund Freud.

179 **True** Animus is the unconscious masculine side of the woman's female persona.

180 **False** According to Adler, 'inferiority complex' is concerned with specific body organs either in reality or in fantasy.

181 **False** The concept of 'transitional object' is associated with Winnicott. It is an intermediate between eroticism and true object relationships.

182 **False** The concept of free association is associated with Sigmund Freud.

183 **True** Persona is the front we present to the world.

184 **True** Anima is the unconscious feminine side of the man's male persona.

185 **False** It is associated with Melanie Klein. It is the realization that the mother is both good and bad which leads to guilt and fear of destroying loved ones with hatred.

186 **False**

187 **False**

188 **True**

189 **True**

190 **True**

191 **True** According to psychoanalytic theory, anxiety is viewed as the result of 'psychic conflict' between unconscious sexual or aggressive wishes stemming from the id and corresponding threats of punishment from the superego.

Clinical theory and skills

Aetiology

192 **True** It is proposed that anxiety is experienced for the first time during the process of birth (primary anxiety).

193 **False** It is linked with depression.

194 **True** During the oedipal phase, anxiety focuses on potential damage to or loss of the genitals of a retaliatory parental figure.

195 **True** It is thought that the child is overwhelmed by stimulation at the very moment of separation from its mother. It has been suggested that this may explain why separation can provoke anxiety.

196 **False**   It is linked with depression. Anxiety is an affect that was instrumental in the birth of psychoanalysis and psychodynamic psychiatry. Freud considered anxiety as both a symptomatic manifestation of neurotic conflict as well as an adaptive signal to ward off awareness of neurotic conflict.

197 **True**

198 **True**

199 **True**

200 **True**

201 **False**   Learning is a relatively permanent change in behaviour brought about as a result of prior experience. Learning may occur through associations being made between two or more phenomena. There are three types of learning theory: associative learning (classical and operant conditioning), cognitive learning and social learning.

202 **True**

203 **True**

204 **True**

205 **True**

Diagnosis/classification

206 **True**

207 **False**   It is an axis II diagnosis.

208 **False**

209 **True**

210 **False**   There is no separate category of late paraphrenia under schizophrenia and other psychotic disorders.

211 **False**   The main feature of somatoform disorder is repeated presentation of the physical symptom together with persistent requests for medical investigations, in spite of repeated negative findings and reassurances by doctors that the symptoms have no physical basis.

212 **True**   It is a rare disorder, characterized by the 'approximate answers' usually accompanied by dissociative symptoms.

213 **False**   Neurasthenia is characterized by either the persistent and distressing complaints of increased fatigue after mental effort or the same complaints of bodily weakness and exhaustion after a minimal physical effort.

214 **True**   It is a rare disorder characterized by the apparent evidence of two or more distinct personalities within an individual with only one of them being evident at a given time.

215 **False**   Essential features of hypochondriasis include persistent preoccupation with the possibility of having one or more serious and progressive physical diseases.

216 **True**

217 **False**   In multiaxial classification, the clinical syndrome is recorded on axis I. Other axes allow the systematic recording of different information sets.

218 **True**

219 **True**

220 **False**   Diagnostic reliability is considerably higher using structured and standardized interviews than is possible with unstructured interviews.

History taking/interviewing

221 **False**

222 **True**

223 **True**

224 False

225 **True**   Open-ended questions encourage the patient to mention his or her main problems. The interviewer should begin history taking by asking an open-ended question.

226 **False**

227 **True**

228 **True**

229 **False**

230 **False**   Before the interview begins, the interviewer should ensure that the patient knows the purpose of the interview and that the setting is right.

231 **True**

232 **True**

233 **False**   Standardized rating scales are useful but not necessary in day-to-day clinical practice.

234 **False**   During an interview, the patient may give hints of important problems or feelings by changes in tone, facial expression or posture. The interviewer should be alert to this possibility and pursue such cues by commenting on them.

235 **True**

236 **False**

237 **True**

238 **False**

239 **False**

240 **False**

Mental state examination

241 **True**

242 **True**

243 **False**

244 **False**

245 **False**

246 **False**

247 **False**

248 **True**

249 **True**

250 **False**

Physical/neurological examination

251 **True**

252 **True**

253 **True**

254 **False** It may also occur with lesions of the dominant temporal lobe.

255 **False** See answer 254. The other features include hemisomatognosia, prosopagnosia, psychotic symptomatology and convulsions. However, the last two symptoms are not specific to lesions of the non-dominant temporal lobe.

256 **True** Wernicke's encephalopathy is caused by deficiency of thiamine (vitamin B_1). The other features include ophthalmoplegia and clouding of consciousness.

257 **True**

258 **False**

259 **True**

260 **False** It is associated with vitamin B_{12} deficiency.

PAPER 5 ISQs

Questions

Basic sciences

Basic psychology

1   Short-term memory process is normally subjected to interference.

2   Short-term memory has a limited capacity for storage of information.

3   Short-term memory process is selective in the material that is retained.

4   Acting out is most commonly manifested by aggressive behaviour towards the self.

5   Minnesota Multiphasic Personality Inventory is a projective test of personality.

6   Retrieval of memorized information is improved by being in the context as and when that information was learnt.

7   Retrieval of memorized information is improved by visual imagery during encoding.

8   Retrieval of memorized information early in a word list is known as the 'primacy effect'.

9   Word Association Technique is useful in assessing personality profile.

10   Rorschach's test is an objective test of personality.

11   The term 'instinctual behaviour' refers to pre-programmed and unlearnt behaviour.

12   Short-term memory has an unlimited capacity to store new information.

13   The term 'attribution theory' refers to a cognitive approach concerned with how people perceive the causes of their behaviour.

14   According to attribution theory, people are likely to attribute their behaviour to their personality traits.

15   According to attribution theory, it is unwise to describe a desired effect of a drug as very strong because the patients may believe that it is the only reason they got better.

16   The term 'learned helplessness' is used to describe the situation where an organism learns that by changing its behaviour it can control the environment.

17   The term 'cognition' refers to the process of obtaining, organizing and using intellectual knowledge.

18   The term 'cognition' refers to an understanding of connection between cause and effect, and between action and its consequences.

19   According to the theory of cognitive learning, cognitive strategies are mental plans to understand other people's behaviour and their environment.

20   The intensity of motivation to achieve any task in a particular situation is determined by at least four factors, such as achievement motive.

[answers on page 137]

Behavioural psychology

21   When assessing a patient for behaviour therapy, operational definitions are used for behaviour patterns.

22   When assessing a patient for behaviour therapy, functional analysis of behaviour is an absolute necessity.

23   When assessing a patient for behaviour therapy, quantitative rating of behaviour is routinely done.

24   When assessing a patient for behaviour therapy, associated cognitions are generally ignored.

25   In behaviour therapy, the schedules of reinforcement are intermittent.

26   With regard to the cognitive theory explanation of panic disorder, the initial attack is a *de novo* event.

27   With regard to the cognitive theory explanation of panic disorder, subsequent avoidance plays a part in maintaining the panic attacks.

28   With regard to the cognitive theory explanation of panic disorder, the panic attacks occur in response to external stimuli.

29   With regard to the cognitive theory explanation of panic disorder, anxiety attacks in childhood contribute greatly to its reoccurrence in adult life.

30   With regard to the cognitive theory explanation of panic disorder, bodily sensations are misinterpreted as being indicative of an underlying physical illness.

31   A functional behavioural analysis uses a subjective account of the antecedents of the problem by the patient.

32   A functional behavioural analysis uses the assumption that immediate consequences are the key determinant of behaviour.

33   A functional behavioural analysis includes an operational definition of the behaviour.

34   A functional behavioural analysis aims to define the problem and identify key variables.

35   A functional behavioural analysis consists of a highly detailed account of predisposing factors.

[answers on page 137]

Neuropsychology

36   The Halstead–Reitan Neurological Battery includes Wechsler's Adult Intelligence Scale.

37   The Trail Making Test assesses visual scanning and visuomotor coordination.

38   Speech Sound Perception Test is used to assess parietal lobe function.

[answers on page 138]

Human development

39   Stranger anxiety is a reflection of insecure attachment.

40   Stranger anxiety is a differentiation of self from the mother.

41   According to Bowlby, most infants by the end of the first 6 months have a hierarchy of attachment figures.

42   According to Margaret Mahler, the framework of normal and deviant development includes a sequence of protest, despair and detachment.

43   According to Margaret Mahler, the framework of normal and deviant development includes the development of object relations within the basic structure of psychoanalytic theory.

44   Fear of falling from a height regularly occurs in the first year of life.

45   Fear of darkness regularly occurs in the first year of life.

46   According to the fundamental assumptions of life cycle theories, human development occurs in clearly defined successive stages.

47   The transitional object represents the transition from inner to outer reality.

48   Attachment behaviour in early childhood is derived predominantly from parental reinforcement.

49   A large family with four or more children is likely to be associated with antisocial behaviour in boys.

50   Studies of childhood fears in the general population indicate that irrational anxieties are rare among children.

[answers on page 138]

Psychopharmacology

General principles

51   Placebo effect in a clinical drug trial refers to the tendency to react to the shape and size of the drug presentation.

52   Placebo effect in a clinical drug trial refers to the tendency to improve on the basis of expectancy and mental attitude even to dummy preparations.

53   Placebo effect in a clinical drug trial refers to a superficial and short-lived response to an active drug preparation.

54   Placebo effect in a clinical drug trial refers to the tendency to respond to the colour of the drug preparation.

55   Placebo effect in a clinical drug trial refers to worsening of a patient's condition in the placebo group.

[answers on page 138]

Pharmacokinetics

56   With regard to the pharmacokinetics of drugs, the therapeutic window is the range of plasma concentration, which yields therapeutic success.

57   Risperidone has a first-dose hypotensive effect due to alpha-1 adrenergic blockade.

58   The pharmacological basis of dopamine-related hypersalivation includes muscarinic M_4 agonism.

59   The pharmacological basis of dopamine-related hypersalivation includes alpha-2 adrenergic antagonism.

60   The pharmacological basis of clozapine-related hypersalivation includes inhibition of the swallowing reflex.

61   Olanzapine causes dose-dependent transient hyperprolactinaemia.

62   Diabetes mellitus associated with clozapine is usually linked to a family history of the same.

63   Diabetes mellitus associated with clozapine is usually linked to obesity.

64   With reference to the effects of antipsychotic drugs on cognition, long-term treatment does not cause any significant impairment on psychometric tests.

65   With reference to the effects of antipsychotic drugs on cognition, impairment of memory is attributed to nigrostriatal dopamine blockade.

[answers on page 139]

Pharmacodynamics

66   With regard to receptor ligands, competitive antagonists block the effects of both agonists and antagonists.

67   With regard to receptor ligands, flumazenil is an antagonist with potential inverse agonist effects.

68   Drugs, which selectively block potassium channels, may have therapeutic uses in patients with multiple sclerosis.

69   The D_2 dopamine receptor inhibits the activity of adenylate cyclase.

70   Presynaptic inhibition is restricted to noradrenergic and GABAergic synapses.

71   With regard to psychotropic drugs, D_2 receptor agonists possess antipsychotic activity.

72   With regard to psychotropic drugs, amitriptyline causes dry mouth by antagonism of muscarinic receptors.

73   With regard to psychotropic drugs, lorazepam opens up chloride channels, which enhance GABA transmission.

74   With regard to psychotropic drugs, lithium primarily acts by blocking reuptake of catecholamines.

75   With regard to psychotropic drugs, buspirone antagonizes 5-hydroxytryptamine (5-HT) receptors.

[answers on page 139]

Adverse drug reactions

76   The adverse effect of persistent fine tremors requires immediate discontinuation of lithium.

77   The adverse effect of ataxia requires immediate discontinuation of lithium.

78   The adverse effect of slurred speech requires immediate discontinuation of lithium.

79   The adverse effect of persistent polyuria and polydipsia requires immediate discontinuation of lithium.

80   The adverse effect of muscular weakness requires immediate discontinuation of lithium.

81 Abrupt withdrawal of a tricyclic antidepressant drug is followed by relapse of depression.

82 Abrupt withdrawal of a tricyclic antidepressant drug may be followed by nausea.

83 Vomiting follows abrupt withdrawal of a tricyclic antidepressant drug.

84 Abrupt withdrawal of a tricyclic antidepressant drug is followed by anxiety.

85 Abrupt withdrawal of a tricyclic antidepressant drug may be followed by convulsions.

86 Ataxia is a characteristic feature of a neurotoxic reaction.

87 Nystagmus is a characteristic feature of a neurotoxic reaction.

88 Hyporeflexia is a characteristic feature of a neurotoxic reaction.

89 Psychomotor retardation is a characteristic feature of a neurotoxic reaction.

90 Extensor plantar response is a characteristic feature of a neurotoxic reaction.

91 Euphoria is a recognized unwanted effect of antimuscarinic drugs.

92 Dry mouth is a recognized unwanted effect of antimuscarinic drugs.

93 Insomnia is a recognized unwanted effect of antimuscarinic drugs.

94 Constipation is a recognized unwanted effect of antimuscarinic drugs.

95 Drowsiness is a recognized unwanted effect of antimuscarinic drugs.

[answers on page 140]

Psychopathology

Descriptive

96 Pareidolia is a characteristic feature of patients with schizophrenia.

97 Omission is a characteristic feature of patients with schizophrenia.

98 Clang associations are characteristic features of patients with schizophrenia.

99 Audible thoughts are characteristic features of patients with schizophrenia.

100 Derailment is a characteristic feature of patients with schizophrenia.

101 Ruminations are characteristically distressing.

102 Ruminations are usually associated with rituals.

103   Ruminations are often resisted but not acted upon.

104   Ruminations are usually considered prodromal symptoms of schizophrenia.

105   Ruminations are considered to be a normal experience.

106   Sublimation is a prominent defence mechanism found in conversion disorders.

107   Sublimation is associated with fixation at the oral stage.

108   Sublimation is a neurotic ego defence mechanism.

109   Sublimation involves diversion of immediate gratification to something else.

110   Sublimation means diversion of unacceptable impulses to acceptable outlets.

111   Patients with a fear of blushing usually avoid well-lit rooms.

112   Patients with a fear of blushing often suffer from social phobia.

113   Patients with a fear of blushing are vulnerable when they are bored.

114   Patients with a fear of blushing will often feign a toothache.

115   Patients with a fear of blushing often abuse alcohol.

116   Perseveration is a disorder of form of speech.

117   Pressure of speech is a disorder of form of speech.

118   Psychomotor retardation is a disorder of form of speech.

119   Confabulation is a disorder of form of speech.

120   Flight of ideas is a disorder of form of speech.

121   Near-death experiences are a type of normal human experience.

122   Pseudohallucinations are a type of normal human experience.

123   Ideas of reference are a type of normal human experience.

124   Panoramic memory is a type of normal human experience.

125   Delusional mood is a type of normal human experience.

126   Auditory hallucinations are a type of abnormal perception.

127   Gustatory hallucinations are a type of normal perception.

128   Complex visual hallucinations are a type of normal perception.

129   Hypnagogic hallucinations are a type of normal perception.

130   Hypnopompic hallucinations are a type of abnormal perception.

131   Catalepsy is an example of a dissociative state.

132   Somnambulism is an example of a dissociative state.

133   Night terrors are an example of a dissociative state.

134   Cataplexy is an example of a dissociative state.

135   Hysterical amnesia is an example of a dissociative state.

136   Withdrawal from social contacts is a typical feature of schizoid personality.

137   Avoidance of competitive situations is a typical feature of schizoid personality.

138   Typical features of schizoid personality include intemperate outbursts of anger.

139   A tendency to distort friendly actions of others as hostile is a typical feature of schizoid personality.

140   Tenacious sense of personal rights is a typical feature of schizoid personality.

141   Capgras' syndrome is allied to dissociative states.

142   Capgras' syndrome is also called pure erotomania.

143   Capgras' syndrome is allied to free association.

144   Capgras' syndrome is characterized by delusions of double.

145   Capgras' syndrome is usually associated with paranoid schizophrenia.

[answers on page 140]

Dynamic psychopathology

146   The defence mechanism of denial is significantly associated with dissociative states.

147   The defence mechanism of reaction formation is significantly associated with obsessive–compulsive disorder.

148   The defence mechanism of projective identification is significantly associated with paranoia.

149   The defence mechanism of introjection is significantly associated with pathological grief reaction.

150   The defence mechanism of turning in on oneself is significantly associated with depression.

151   In dynamic psychopathology, 'epinosic gain' is usually secondary to intrapsychic conflicts.

152 In dynamic psychopathology, 'epinosic gain' results in control of anxiety.

153 In dynamic psychopathology, 'epinosic gain' may result in control over people important to the patient.

154 In dynamic psychopathology, 'epinosic gain' is a simultaneous expression of drives and defences.

155 With regard to dynamic psychopathology, 'epinosic gain' assists maintenance of symptoms.

156 With regard to dynamic psychopathology, the working alliance is based on childhood relationships that have enabled the patient to develop basic trust.

157 With regard to dynamic psychopathology, the working alliance is a neurotic, irrational but reasonable rapport between the patient and the therapist.

158 With regard to dynamic psychopathology, the working alliance enables the patient to undergo psychoanalysis despite the transference impulses.

159 With regard to dynamic psychopathology, the working alliance makes it possible for the patient to achieve an insight into her or his problems.

160 With regard to dynamic psychopathology, the working alliance refers to the counter transference relationship with the patient.

161 With regard to psychodynamic concepts, the term 'schizoid' means a preschizophrenic state.

162 With regard to psychodynamic concepts, the term 'schizoid' means being unable to verbalize feelings.

163 With regards to psychodynamic concepts, the term 'schizoid' means being detached, aloof and humourless.

164 With regard to psychodynamic concepts, the term 'schizoid' means a diffuse identity.

165 With regard to psychodynamic concepts, the term 'schizoid' means spilling of the self.

166 The ego is responsible for the interests of the person as a whole.

167 The ego is in a dependent relationship to the claims of the id.

168 The ego is a concept originally used by Melanie Klein.

169 The ego is an expression of the defensive pole of the personality in a neurotic conflict.

170 The ego is essentially reality oriented.

171   The ego is the psychic representation of adaptation to the demands of drives and to the requirements of external reality.

172   The superego is the psychic representation of judgement, self-criticism and conscience.

173   The superego is affectively regulated by guilt.

174   The ego ideal is a component of the superego, which is affectively regulated by shame.

175   The ego is the agent of the personality system that mediates between the demands of the id and the superego.

176   The ego mediates between the personality system and external reality.

177   Primary process thinking is present in patients with psychotic disorders.

[answers on page 143]

Clinical theory and skills

Aetiology

178   Excess of life events prior to the onset of an illness is known to be of aetiological importance in schizophrenia.

179   Having a schizophrenogenic mother is known to be of aetiological importance in schizophrenia.

180   Double-bind communication is known to be of aetiological importance in schizophrenia.

181   Decreased dopamine in mesolimbic tract is known to be of aetiological importance in schizophrenia.

182   Excess of perinatal complications is known to be of aetiological importance in schizophrenia.

183   The processes involved in the maintenance of bulimia nervosa include an over-concern about body shape and body weight.

184   The processes involved in the maintenance of bulimia nervosa include the binges that are perpetuated by continued dieting.

185   The processes involved in the maintenance of bulimia nervosa include frequent purgative and diuretic misuse.

186   The processes involved in the maintenance of bulimia nervosa include the undermining of the patient's self-control and self-esteem.

187   The processes involved in the maintenance of bulimia nervosa include masked depression.

188   Dysmnesic syndrome of recent origin may result from carbon dioxide
       poisoning.

189   Dysmnesic syndrome of recent origin may result from carbon monoxide
       poisoning.

190   Dysmnesic syndrome of recent origin may result from excessive
       consumption of amphetamines.

191   Dysmnesic syndrome of recent origin may result from nicotinic acid
       deficiency.

192   Dysmnesic syndrome of recent origin may result from ingestion of
       lysergic acid diethylamide.

[answers on page 144]

Classification/diagnosis

193   The International Classification of Diseases (ICD)-10 was developed by
       the United Nations in 1992.

194   The ICD-10 is a type of categorical classification.

195   The ICD-10 contains only mental disorders.

196   The ICD-10 was developed by the World Health Organization in 1992.

197   In the ICD-10, the traditional division between neurosis and psychosis is
       retained.

198   The operational criteria for the diagnosis of schizophrenia are included
       in the Diagnostic and Statistical Manual (DSM)-IV.

199   The operational criteria for the diagnosis of schizophrenia include
       Schneider's first rank symptoms.

200   The operational criteria for the diagnosis of schizophrenia are included
       in the ICD-10.

201   The operational criteria for the diagnosis of schizophrenia include
       Bleuler's fundamental and accessory symptoms.

202   The operational criteria for the diagnosis of schizophrenia are included
       in Research Diagnostic Criteria.

203   The DSM-IV is an atheoretical classification.

204   The main text of the DSM-IV does not include classification on
       'neurosis'.

205   The DSM-IV uses operational criteria throughout its text.

206   The DSM-IV retains two kinds of hierarchy of mental disorders.

207   The DSM-IV is a typical example of a multiaxial classification.

208 With regard to the relative merits of categorical classification, it makes it easy to describe the mental disorders.

209 With regard to the relative merits of categorical classification, the disorders, which lie halfway between two disorders, are given special attention.

210 With regard to the relative merits of categorical classification, it is a more flexible system than dimensional classification.

211 With regard to the relative merits of categorical classification, it is based in aetiological factors.

212 With regard to the relative merits of categorical classification, it does not strain the resources of a conservative and largely innumerate profession.

[answers on page 145]

History taking/interviewing

213 With regard to the initial assessment of a psychotic patient, one should confidently confront the psychotic symptoms.

214 With regard to the initial assessment of a psychotic patient, colluding with paranoid delusions is a wise step.

215 With regard to the initial assessment of a psychotic patient, the clinician must be careful to avoid implying any expectations in his or her questions.

216 With regard to the initial assessment of a psychotic patient, it is sensible to enquire about psychotic symptomatology first before asking screening questions in other areas.

217 With regard to the initial assessment of a psychotic patient, mental state examination may reveal useful information before taking a full history.

218 With regard to the initial assessment of a patient who abuses alcohol, the family members should be involved at this stage.

219 With regard to the initial assessment of a patient who abuses alcohol, the therapeutic goals should be set at the outset.

220 With regard to the initial assessment of a patient who abuses alcohol, enquiries should be made about trouble with police.

221 With regard to the initial assessment of a patient who abuses alcohol, the CAGE questionnaire should be applied to identify at risk drinkers.

222 With regard to the initial assessment of a patient who abuses alcohol, enquiry about the time of the first drink of the day is important.

223 With regard to psychiatric history taking, sometimes a detailed history should be taken after the mental state examination.

224 With regard to psychiatric history taking, during the first few minutes, the patient should be allowed to talk freely about whatever he or she wants to express.

225 With regard to psychiatric history taking, direct questions should never be asked.

226 With regard to psychiatric history taking, the interview should begin by explaining the exact purpose of the interview.

227 With regard to psychiatric history taking, non-verbal clues are as important as verbal clues.

228 Rapid cycling bipolar affective disorder is defined as four or more episodes of depression, mania or hypomania in the previous 12 months.

229 'Normality' between an episode of mania and an episode of depression is not required to make a diagnosis of rapid cycling affective disorder.

230 In rapid cycling bipolar affective disorder, episodes are demarcated by a switch to an episode of opposite polarity or a period of remission.

[answers on page 145]

Mental state examination

231 Lack of selective inattention is implicated in behavioural patterns occurring in dissociative states.

232 Lack of selective inattention is implicated in behavioural patterns occurring in Alzheimer's disease.

233 Lack of selective inattention is implicated in behavioural patterns seen in patients with depression.

234 Lack of selective inattention is implicated in behavioural patterns seen in patients with schizophrenia.

235 Lack of selective inattention is implicated in behavioural patterns seen in patients with anorexia nervosa.

[answers on page 146]

Physical/neurological examination

236 Abnormal voluntary movements typically occur in tardive dyskinesia.

237 Abnormal voluntary movements typically occur in echopraxia.

238 Abnormal voluntary movements typically occur in Alzheimer's disease.

239 Abnormal voluntary movements typically occur in Parkinson's disease.

240   Abnormal voluntary movements typically occur in chronic schizophrenia.

241   Indications for a computed tomography (CT) scan include a suspicion of a cerebral tumour.

242   Indications for a CT scan include a suspicion of subdural haematoma.

243   Indications for a CT scan include presence of focal neurological signs.

244   Indications for a CT scan include clinical pointers of normal-pressure hydrocephalus.

245   Indications for a CT scan include cerebral oedema.

246   Amnesia is a recognized feature of motor neurone disease.

247   Dysarthria is a recognized feature of motor neurone disease.

248   Dysphagia is a recognized feature of motor neurone disease.

249   Intention tremor is a recognized feature of motor neurone disease.

250   Uncontrollable laughter is a recognized feature of motor neurone disease.

251   Lesions of the caudate nucleus are associated with significant memory loss.

252   Lesions of the substantia innominata are associated with significant memory loss.

253   Lesions of the anterior nucleus of the thalamus are associated with significant memory loss.

254   Lesions of the hypothalamus are associated with significant memory loss.

255   Lesions of the globus pallidus are associated with significant memory loss.

256   Spasmodic torticollis in a 30- to 50-year-old man is almost always psychogenic in origin.

257   Spasmodic torticollis in a 30- to 50-year-old man responds to behaviour therapy.

258   Spasmodic torticollis in a 30- to 50-year-old man may be a presenting symptom of Parkinson's disease.

259   Spasmodic torticollis in a 30- to 50-year-old man requires surgical correction.

260   Spasmodic torticollis in a 30- to 50-year-old man is certainly psychogenic if the patient can abolish it temporarily by touching the face on the affected side.

[answers on page 146]

Answers and explanations

Basic sciences

Basic psychology

1   True
2   True
3   False
4   False
5   False
6   True
7   True
8   False
9   True
10 False
11 True
12 False
13 True
14 False   People are likely to attribute their behaviour to situational causes but are likely to attribute others' behaviour to stable internal dispositions, i.e. personality traits.
15 True
16 False   It is used to explain depression in human beings who feel helpless, without options and unable to control events.
17 True
18 True
19 True
20 False

Behavioural psychology

21 False
22 True
23 True
24 True
25 True   Other schedules of reinforcement include continuous reinforcement, mixed interval, variable interval, mixed ratio and variable ratio reinforcement. In behaviour therapy, emphasis is placed not on diagnosing syndromes, but on discovering current factors related to the problem. The treatment is only given after a detailed examination of the precise circumstances surrounding the problem, i.e. functional behavioural analysis.
26 False   Although cognitive theory does not specifically address the first attack, it is thought that most panic attacks occur as a result of a tendency to catastrophically misinterpret bodily sensations.

27   **True**   Avoidance helps by reinforcing the person's belief that something disastrous was prevented from happening by his or her actions.
28   **False**   Any stimulus that is perceived as threatening either external or internal can lead to a panic attack.
29   **False**
30   **False**   Although to an extent this response may seem correct, the crucial factor is the person believing that something catastrophic is about to happen immediately.
31   **True**
32   **True**
33   **False**   It includes the subject's overt responses such as avoidance, escape and ritualistic behaviours. Operational definitions of these responses are not usually included.
34   **True**
35   **False**   It consists of a highly detailed account of current determinants of the problem. Behaviour therapy is interested in the perpetuating factors.

Neuropsychology

36   **True**   It also includes MMPI and Trail making and Category Tests.
37   **True**
38   **False**   It is a test of temporal lobe functions.

Human development

39   **False**
40   **True**
41   **True**
42   **False**
43   **True**
44   **True**
45   **True**
46   **True**
47   **True**
48   **False**
49   **True**
50   **False**

Psychopharmacology

General principles

51   **True**
52   **True**
53   **False**
54   **True**

55 **False** The placebo effect refers to the fact that any treatment will produce beneficial results if given or taken with enough faith and enthusiasm. It is dependent on a number of factors such as the nature and quantity of the placebo preparation given, the situation and the manner in which it is given, the social and psychological attributes of the recipient, the condition being treated, etc.

Pharmacokinetics

56 **True**
57 **True**
58 **True**
59 **True**
60 **True**
61 **True**
62 **False**
63 **False**
64 **True**
65 **False** It is attributed to antimuscarinic effects.

Pharmacodynamics

66 **False** They block the effects of agonists and inverse agonists.
67 **True** Flumazenil is an antagonist to diazepam and has slight partial inverse agonist effects, leading to anxiogenic features in patients with panic attacks.
68 **True**
69 **True** D_1 receptors stimulate and D_2 receptors inhibit adenyl cyclase.
70 **False** Presynaptic inhibition occurs in noradrenergic and GABAergic synapses and also in dopaminergic and serotonergic synapses.
71 **False** D_2 receptor antagonists are believed to possess antipsychotic activity.
72 **True**
73 **False** Benzodiazepines act directly by binding with benzodiazepine receptors, which are themselves linked to gamma-aminobutyric acid (GABA) receptors in an ionophore or complex involving GABA, benzodiazepine receptors and chloral channels. In addition, they block cortical arousal, which occurs after stimulation of the midbrain reticular activating system.
74 **False** Its mode of action in the treatment of affective disorders has not been identified. It is postulated that lithium stimulates sodium and magnesium-dependent adenosine triphosphatase (ATPase). It inhibits adenyl cyclase and inositol phosphate intracellular secondary messenger systems throughout the body. It also alters the functions of guanosine triphosphate (GTP)-binding proteins.
75 **False** Its action appears to be mediated through 5-HT_{1A} receptors, where it is a partial agonist, and D_2 receptors to which it weakly binds.

Adverse drug reactions

76   False

77   True

78   True

79   False

80   True   Signs of lithium intoxication include blurred vision, increasing gastrointestinal disturbances (anorexia, vomiting and diarrhoea), coarse tremor, and lack of coordination, dysarthria, nystagmus and convulsions. Lithium should be stopped immediately, serum lithium concentration redetermined and steps taken to reverse lithium toxicity.

81   False

82   True

83   False

84   False

85   False   A few patients, who are accustomed to a fairly high dose of a tricyclic antidepressant drug, will experience a withdrawal syndrome if the drug is abruptly withdrawn. This syndrome is characterized by malaise, headache, nausea, abdominal pain, diarrhoea, and restlessness. It is characterized by cholinergic hyperfunction.

86   True

87   True

88   True

89   True

90   False   Neurotoxic effects may be acute or chronic. Potential mechanisms include selective interference with basic metabolic processes, protein and nucleic acid synthesis, nerve membrane permeability or synaptic transmission. The clinical picture includes symptoms of severe motor, mental and autonomic disorders.

91   True

92   True

93   True

94   True

95   True   Antimuscarinic drugs exert their antiparkinsonian effect by correcting the relative central cholinergic excess thought to occur in Parkinsonism as a result of dopamine deficiency. Their unwanted effects include gastrointestinal disturbances, dizziness, blurred vision, urinary retention, tachycardia, nervousness and excitement.

Psychopathology

Descriptive

96   False   Pareidolia is a type of illusion in which real and unreal percepts exist side by side, the latter being recognized as unreal. It occurs in normal people and also in acute organic brain disorder.

97   True   It consists of senseless omission of a thought or part of it.

98 **True** Clang associations refer to words with similar sounds, which are used to preserve the ordinary logical sequence of ideas. They occur in poetry, humour and manic episodes.

99 **True** It is a Schneider's first rank symptom in which the patient hears his or her own thoughts out loud. The patient knows that the thoughts are their own.

100 **True** It is a type of loosening of associations. It refers to a transition from one topic to another, either between sentences or mid-sentence with no logical relation between two topics. It is also known as Knight's move.

101 **True** Obsessional ruminations are repeated worrying themes of a complex kind, e.g. about ending of the world.

102 **True** Rituals, i.e. compulsions, are usually associated with obsessions if they have the function of reducing the distress caused by the latter.

103 **False** This refers to compulsive rituals.

104 **False** A prodrome of non-specific symptoms appears in some young people. It includes symptoms such as loss of interest, avoiding the company of others, staying away from work, irritability and oversensitivity.

105 **True**

106 **False** Sublimation is a mature or healthy ego defence mechanism.

107 **False** It is associated with the latency phase of psychosexual development.

108 **False** See answer 106.

109 **False**

110 **True**

111 **False** The essential feature of social phobia is a marked and persistent fear of social or performance situations in which embarrassment may occur.

112 **True** The other symptoms of social phobia include palpitations, tremors, sweating, gastrointestinal discomfort, diarrhoea, muscle tension and confusion.

113 **False** The patient typically avoids the feared situations.

114 **False**

115 **True** Some patients take alcohol to relieve the symptoms of anxiety. Alcohol abuse is more common in patients suffering from social phobias than other phobias.

116 **False** Perseveration usually occurs in association with disturbance of memory. It is defined as a response that was appropriate to a first stimulus being given inappropriately to a second, different stimulus.

117 **False** It is a disorder of the stream of thought. Here ideas arise in unusual variety and abundance. They pass through the mind rapidly.

118 **False** It is a disorder of stream of thought. Here the patient has only a few thoughts, which lack variety and richness. They move through the mind slowly.

119 **False** Confabulation is a falsification of memory occurring in clear consciousness in association with an organically derived amnesia.

120 **False** It is a disorder of tempo of thinking in which there is no general direction of thinking. The connections between successive thoughts appear to be due to chance factors, which usually are understood.

121 **True** Near-death experience is a complex hallucinatory phenomenon in people who perceive death as imminent. It seems to be comparable to other mental reactions to perceived threat, coloured by culture and current stress.

122 **True** Pseudohallucinations are a type of mental image, which although clear and vivid lack the substantiality of perceptions. They are seen in full consciousness, known not to be real perceptions. They are located in the person's subjective space.

123 **True** People who are usually self-conscious hold ideas of reference. The person realizes that this feeling originates within him- or herself. They are present in many mental disorders.

124 **True**

125 **True** In delusional mood, the patient has the knowledge that there is something strange going around him or her, which concerns the person; they do not know what it is. Usually the meaning of delusional mood becomes apparent when a sudden delusional perception occurs.

126 **True**

127 **False**

128 **False**

129 **False**

130 **True** Abnormal perceptions are divided into: (i) sensory distortions where a real perceptual object is perceived distorted, and (ii) false perceptions, where new perceptions occur which may or may not be in response to external stimuli, e.g. illusions and hallucinations.

131 **False** Catalepsy is a disorder of muscle tone in which the patient allows him or herself to be placed in an awkward posture which he or she maintains apparently without distress much longer than most people could achieve without severe discomfort.

132 **True** Somnambulism, i.e. sleep walking usually occurs in children and in males more often than females. Activity is usually confined to aimless wandering and purposeless repetitive behaviour for a few minutes.

133 **False** Night terrors occur in deep sleep early in the night, and often in an individual who also sleep walks. Intense anxiety is manifested. Usually, there is amnesia for the experience on waking.

134 **False** In cataplexy, the subject falls due to sudden loss of muscle tone provoked by strong emotions.

135 **True** The common theme shared by dissociative states is a partial or complete loss of normal integration between memories of the past, awareness of identity and immediate sensations and control of bodily movements. Dissociative states tend to remit after a few weeks or months.

136 **True**

137 **True**

138 **False** The patient has limited capacity to express either warm, tender feelings, or anger towards others.

139 **False** The patient is apparently indifferent to either praise or criticism.

140 **False** The patient exhibits excessive preoccupation with fantasy and introspection. He or she also shows marked insensitivity to prevailing social norms and conventions.

141 **False**

142 **False**

143 **False** Free association is a psychoanalytic technique.

144 **True**

145 **True** Capgras and Reboul–Lachaux, first described Capgras' syndrome in 1923. It is strictly speaking a single symptom and not a syndrome; namely that a person closely related to the patient has been replaced by an identical double. The patient accepts that the misidentified person has a great resemblance to the familiar person, but still they are different people. It is also associated with affective and organic disorders.

Dynamic psychopathology

146 **True**

147 **True**

148 **False**

149 **True**

150 **True**

151 **False** The term 'epinosic' means secondary to an illness, i.e. it refers to a secondary gain.

152 **False** The control of anxiety is in fact a primary gain. However, the patient may exercise considerable control over the environment and the people around him or her.

153 **True**

154 **True**

155 **True**

156 **True**

157 **False** The patient's relationship with the therapist is a mixture of a transference relationship and a real relationship. This latter relationship is termed as a therapeutic or working alliance. As part of the working alliance, the patient must achieve a realistic view of the treatment programme.

158 **True**

159 **True**

160 **False** See answer 157.

161 **False**

162 **True**

163 **True**

164 **True**

165 **True** From a psychodynamic perspective, the term 'schizoid' reflects a splitting or fragmentation of the self into different self-representations that remain unintegrated. The result is a diffuse identity, i.e. the schizoid persons are not sure who they are.

166 **True**   The ego corresponds to the conscious level of functioning. It develops progressively from birth. Its first task is to distinguish between the inner world of subjective experience and external reality.

167 **True**

168 **False**   It is a concept used by Freudian analysts.

169 **True**

170 **True**   As ego is reality oriented, it has to find acceptable and appropriate ways of satisfying the demands of id, which may involve delaying its gratification.

171 **True**

172 **True**

173 **True**

174 **True**

175 **True**

176 **True**

177 **True**

Clinical theory and skills

Aetiology

178 **True**   Although life events seem to have an effect, the size of the effect is uncertain.

179 **False**   None of the theories of disordered communication within the family can give a satisfactory explanation why it is unusual for more than one child in a family to develop schizophrenia.

180 **False**   A double-bind is said to occur when an instruction is given overtly but contradicted by a second, more covert instruction.

181 **False**   The dopamine hypothesis indicated that there is a dopamine over activity in the mesolimbic system.

182 **True**   Retrospective studies of schizophrenic patients report more obstetric complications than normal controls.

183 **True**

184 **True**

185 **True**

186 **True**

187 **False**   There are several processes that maintain bulimia nervosa once it is established. Over-concern drives dieting; the dieting in turn is likely to encourage binges, which are also encouraged by the purgatives and diuretic abuse, as well as by self-induced vomiting. The binges undermine the patient's sense of self-control and self-esteem, thus exacerbating feelings of ineffectiveness and intensifying concern with shape and weight.

188 **True**

189 **True**

190 **True**

191 **True**

192 **False**

Classification/diagnosis

193 **False**   It was published by the World Health Organization in 1992.
194 **True**
195 **False**
196 **True**
197 **False**   The traditional division between neurosis and psychosis has not been used but the term 'neurotic' is still retained for occasional use in categories F40–F48.
198 **True**
199 **True**
200 **True**
201 **True**
202 **True**
203 **True**   Most diagnoses have empirical literature or available data sets that are relevant to decisions regarding the revision of the diagnostic manual.
204 **True**
205 **True**
206 **True**   It retains two kinds of hierarchy: organic mental disorder pre-empts the diagnosis of any disorder that could produce part of the symptomatology, and psychotic disorders pre-empt other disorders in the same way.
207 **True**   It involves an assessment on several axes, each of which refers to a different domain of information that may help the clinician plan treatment and predict outcome.
208 **True**
209 **False**   One of the serious drawbacks is that these disorders may be overlooked or misrepresented.
210 **False**   In fact, the dimensional classification system is more flexible than the categorical classification.
211 **False**   It is based on subject matter, which is divided into a number of separate and mutually exclusive categories.
212 **True**

History taking/interviewing

213 **False**   Confrontation with the patient may lead to irritable and uncooperative behaviour on the part of the patient.
214 **False**   One should be neutral in approaching the paranoid delusions.
215 **True**
216 **True**
217 **True**
218 **False**
219 **True**
220 **True**
221 **True**

222 **True** Usually patients who are dependent on alcohol take the first drink in the morning to control tremors, as well as other unpleasant withdrawal symptoms.

223 **True** When the patient is disturbed or has organic brain disease, the mental state is more crucial, as it is not possible to take a history from the patient.

224 **True**

225 **False**

226 **True**

227 **True**

228 **True**

229 **False**

230 **True**

Mental state examination

231 **True** In dissociative states, it is presumed that the ability to exercise conscious and selective control is impaired.

232 **True**

233 **True**

234 **True**

235 **False** Because of limited capacity to our information processing system, it is essential that we are able to restrict the total input to a manageable amount. It is also necessary to ensure that important information is allowed through for processing while the irrelevant and unimportant information is screened out.

Physical/neurological examination

236 **False**

237 **True**

238 **False**

239 **False**

240 **True**

241 **True**

242 **True**

243 **True**

244 **True**

245 **True** CT is used extensively in clinical practice. It is able to demonstrate shifts of intracranial structures and expanding intracranial lesions. It has also proved to be a useful psychiatric research tool.

246 **False**

247 **True**

248 **True**

249 **False**

250 **True** The features of motor neurone disease include difficulty in swallowing, chewing, coughing, breathing and talking, wasted and fasciculating tongue, muscle stiffness and weakness. There are no objective changes on sensory examination.

251 **False**   Caudate nucleus and globus pallidus are principal components of corpus striatum of the basal ganglia. The corpus striatum is important in control of posture and initiation of movement. It is probably involved in the balance between alpha and gamma motor neurone activity.

252 **True**

253 **True**

254 **True**   The hypothalamus acts as a control centre for the regulation of the internal environment.

255 **False**

256 **False**

257 **True**   Where the aetiology is uncertain, it is justifiable to combine physically oriented measures and psychological techniques such as behaviour therapy and psychotherapy.

258 **False**

259 **True**

260 **False**   Spasmodic torticollis is a rare condition in which there are repeated purposeless movements of the head and neck or sustained abnormal positions or both. Its causes include organic and psychological factors.

PAPER 6 ISQs

Questions

Basic sciences

Basic psychology

1   In information processing, selective attention involves filtering.

2   In information processing, selective attention involves concentrating.

3   In information processing, selective attention involves pigeonholing.

4   In information processing, selective attention involves telescoping.

5   In information processing, selective attention involves categorizing.

6   In operant conditioning, when a rat is given a shock in one end of a box and it runs to the other end, the learning process is called 'avoidance training'.

7   In operant conditioning, when a rat presses a lever more often because it obtains food, it is called 'survival training'.

8   In operant conditioning, if a rat responds by running away at the sound of a bell, rung before an electric current is delivered, this is called 'escape training'.

9   In operant conditioning, if a rat is given an electric current with no way of escape or avoidance, it is called 'punitive training'.

10   In operant conditioning, when a rat is given gradually increasing levels of electric current, it is called 'habitual training'.

11   Satisfaction in personal relationships is adversely affected by dysfunctional beliefs such as disagreement is destructive.

12   Wechsler's Adult Intelligence Scale is useful in testing the functions of temporal lobes.

[answers on page 162]

Behavioural psychology

13   In functional behavioural analysis, a history of patient's social relationships is irrelevant.

14   In functional behavioural analysis, clarification of the circumstances that maintain problem behaviour forms an important component.

15 In functional behavioural analysis, the defence mechanisms responsible for the problem behaviour are analysed.

16 In functional behavioural analysis, motivational analysis is included.

17 Observational learning is an important form of learning in childhood.

18 Observational learning includes modelling.

19 Observational learning is an effective treatment for phobias.

20 Observational learning is part of respondent learning.

21 Observational learning requires a behavioural sequence and its consequences to be observed.

22 According to learning theory, negative reinforcement is related to avoidance learning.

23 Negative reinforcement is a process in which a punishment is presented intermittently.

24 According to learning theory, an adventitious reinforcement occurs when responses are accidentally reinforced.

[answers on page 162]

Neuropsychology

25 Grasp reflex is present in adults with parietal lobe dysfunction.

26 Benton visual retention test is useful in testing the functions of the occipital lobe.

27 Testing for apraxias is useful for eliciting frontal lobe dysfunction.

[answers on page 163]

Human development

28 Stranger anxiety is a reaction to the mother's absence.

29 Stranger anxiety is a reflection of object permanence.

30 An example of assimilation in cognitive theory includes an infant smiling preferentially at the sound of his mother's voice.

[answers on page 163]

Psychopharmacology

General principles

31 Citalopram is a non-sedative selective serotonin reuptake inhibitor drug.

32 Moclobemide is a non-sedative antidepressant drug.

33 Sertraline is a non-sedative selective serotonin reuptake inhibitor drug.

34 Paroxetine is a non-sedative selective serotonin reuptake inhibitor drug.

35 Fluoxetine is a non-sedative selective serotonin reuptake inhibitor drug.

36 Loxapine is a type of antipsychotic drug.

37 Pericyazine is a type of antipsychotic drug.

38 Carbamazepine is a type of antipsychotic drug.

39 Fluspirilene is a type of antipsychotic drug.

40 Prochlorperazine is a type of antipsychotic drug.

41 With reference to the effects of antipsychotic drugs, impairment of fine motor coordination is attributed to their antimuscarinic effects.

42 With reference to the effects of antipsychotic drugs, long-term treatment is associated with improvement on most measures of cognition and attention.

43 With reference to the effects of antipsychotic drugs, impairment in cognitive and psychomotor functions occur after acute treatment in patients but not in normal healthy volunteers.

44 Pharmacological treatments are particularly useful in the Gilles de la Tourette syndrome.

45 Pharmacological agents are particularly useful in treating patients exhibiting pica.

46 Pharmacological agents are particularly useful in treating patients exhibiting fire setting.

47 Pharmacological agents are particularly useful in treating patients exhibiting school refusal.

48 Pharmacological agents are particularly useful in treating patients with attention deficit hyperactivity disorder.

49 QT_c values over 500 ms relate to a clearly increased risk of arrhythmia.

[answers on page 163]

Pharmacokinetics

50 QT_c prolongation is most prominent at peak drug plasma levels and least obvious at trough levels.

51 Clozapine appears to increase the plasma levels of insulin in a clozapine-level dependent fashion.

52 The risk of diabetes mellitus has been reported to be higher with atypical antipsychotic drugs than typical drugs with a particular risk in younger patients.

[answers on page 163]

Pharmacodynamics

53   Termination of the neurotransmitter effects in a serotonergic synapse is influenced by reuptake into the postsynaptic membrane.

54   Termination of the neurotransmitter effects in a serotonergic synapse is influenced by monoamine oxidases.

55   Termination of the neurotransmitter effects in a serotonergic synapse is influenced by genomic factors.

56   Termination of the neurotransmitter effects in a serotonergic synapse is influenced by diffusion.

57   Termination of the neurotransmitter effects in a serotonergic synapse is influenced by receptor adaptation.

58   According to current scientific knowledge regarding gamma-aminobutyric acid (GABA) receptors, benzodiazepines occupy a receptor site on the GABA receptor complex.

59   According to current scientific knowledge regarding GABA receptors, glycine acts on the N-methyl-D-aspartate (NMDA) receptors.

60   According to current scientific knowledge regarding GABA receptors, the $GABA_A$ receptor is directly linked to chloride ion channels.

61   According to current scientific knowledge regarding GABA receptors, cyclopyrrolone derivatives increase the frequency of chloride ion channel opening.

62   According to current scientific knowledge regarding GABA receptors, flumazenil blocks the action of agonists on $GABA_B$ receptors.

63   According to current scientific knowledge regarding 5-hydroxytryptamine (5-HT) receptors, 8-hydroxydipropylamine-tetralin (8-OH-DPAT) is a selective agonist of $5-T_{1a}$ receptors.

64   According to current scientific knowledge regarding 5-HT receptors, $5-HT_2$ receptors appear to mediate excitatory effects particularly in the cortex.

65   According to current scientific knowledge, ritanserin is a specific antagonist for $5-HT_2$ receptors.

66   According to current scientific knowledge, ondansetron is a $5-HT_3$ receptor antagonist.

67   According to current scientific knowledge regarding 5-HT receptors, $5-HT_2$ receptors are found in the claustrum, olfactory system and cerebral cortex.

[answers on page 163]

Adverse drug reactions

68   The side effects of tricyclic antidepressant drugs that mimic depressive symptoms include constipation.

69   The side effects of tricyclic antidepressant drugs that mimic depressive symptoms include dry mouth.

70   The side effects of tricyclic antidepressant drugs that mimic depressive symptoms include blurred vision.

71   The side effects of tricyclic antidepressant drugs that mimic depressive symptoms include impaired concentration.

72   The side effects of tricyclic antidepressant drugs that mimic depressive symptoms include black tongue.

73   A patient being treated with a reversible inhibitor of monoamine oxidase (MAO) A should not eat pickled herrings.

74   A patient being treated with a reversible inhibitor of MAO A should not eat aged cheese.

75   A patient being treated with a reversible inhibitor of MAO A should not eat cottage cheese.

76   A patient being treated with a reversible inhibitor of MAO A should not drink red wine.

77   A patient being treated with a reversible inhibitor of MAO A should not eat yeast products.

78   With reference to benzodiazepines, tolerance develops to the ataxic but not to their muscle relaxant properties.

79   With reference to benzodiazepines, tolerance to their anticonvulsant properties develops slowly.

80   With reference to benzodiazepines, tolerance develops to auditory evoked responses.

81   With reference to tolerance to benzodiazepines, tachyphylaxis may develop to their sedative effects.

82   With reference to tolerance to benzodiazepines, it is more likely to develop to their anxiolytic than sedative effects.

83   Hallucinations are common features of benzodiazepine withdrawal syndrome.

84   Seizures are common features of benzodiazepine withdrawal syndrome.

85   Paranoid psychosis is a common feature of benzodiazepine withdrawal syndrome.

86   Confusional states are common features of benzodiazepine withdrawal
      syndrome.

87   Hyperacusis is a common feature of benzodiazepine withdrawal
      syndrome.

[answers on page 164]

Psychopathology

Descriptive

88   Obsessions are sometimes difficult to distinguish from delusions.

89   Obsessions are always recognized by the subjects as being their own
      thoughts.

90   Resistance is a pathognomonic feature of obsessive–compulsive disorder.

91   Obsessions are usually a pleasant experience.

92   Obsessions may present as 'magical thinking'.

93   Alcoholic hallucinosis can present with visual hallucinations.

94   Alcoholic hallucinosis can lead to persecutory delusions.

95   Alcoholic hallucinosis is distinguished from delirium tremens on the
      basis of intact consciousness alone.

96   Alcoholic hallucinosis occurs only after complete discontinuation of
      drinking.

97   A diagnosis of depression is compatible with the presence of obsessions.

98   A diagnosis of depression is compatible with the presence of Schneider's
      first rank symptoms.

99   A diagnosis of depression is compatible with the presence of elated
      mood.

100   A diagnosis of depression is compatible with a past history of
      schizophrenia.

101   A diagnosis of depression is compatible with the presence of alcohol
      dependence.

102   Overdependence on the deceased person is a recognized variable
      adversely affecting the outcome of a grief reaction.

103   Losses that are socially stigmatizing are recognized variables adversely
      affecting the outcome of a grief reaction.

104   Poor prior physical health of the deceased person is a recognized
      variable adversely affecting the outcome of a grief reaction.

105   Loss, which occurs in circumstances where the survivor can be blamed, is a recognized variable adversely affecting the outcome of a grief reaction.

106   Lack of social support is a recognized variable adversely affecting the outcome of a grief reaction.

107   In a manic episode, the diagnosis can only be made in the presence of elated mood.

108   In a manic episode, grandiose delusions are essential clinical features.

109   In a manic episode, decreased attention span suggests an alteration of consciousness.

110   A decreased need for sleep is a useful early warning sign of an impending manic episode.

111   Psychotic features like delusions and hallucinations are more common in mania than depression.

112   Alexithymia is classified under somatoform disorder in the DSM-IV.

113   Beck's Depression Inventory measures alexithymia.

114   Alexithymia refers to people who can describe feelings they do not experience.

115   Alexithymia is usually seen in individuals who are imaginative.

116   Alexithymia is a personality type in which individuals concentrate on their subjective experiences rather than external events.

117   Elated mood can reliably distinguish mania from an acute episode of schizophrenia.

118   Grandiose delusions can reliably distinguish mania from an acute episode of schizophrenia.

119   The presence of Schneider's first rank symptoms can reliably distinguish schizophrenia from mania.

120   Sexually disinhibited behaviour can reliably distinguish mania from an acute episode of schizophrenia.

121   Autochthonous delusions are usually 'ego-dystonic'.

122   Autochthonous delusions are synonymous with delusional perception.

123   The paranoid-schizoid position implies an inability to experience concern for another person.

124   The paranoid-schizoid position implies proneness to primary delusions.

125   The paranoid-schizoid position implies prominent deployment of repression as a defence mechanism.

126   Thought blocking is a negative symptom of schizophrenia.

127   Incongruous affect is a negative symptom of schizophrenia.

128   Avolition is a negative symptom of schizophrenia.

129   Confabulation is a negative symptom of schizophrenia.

130   Psychomotor retardation is a negative symptom of schizophrenia.

131   Spatial disorientation is a recognized feature of puerperal psychosis.

132   Spatial disorientation is a recognized feature of Korsakoff's psychosis.

133   Spatial disorientation is a recognized feature of alcoholic hallucinosis.

134   Spatial disorientation is a recognized feature of Alzheimer's disease.

135   Spatial disorientation is a recognized feature of Ganser's syndrome.

136   Suicide attempters report more life events than patients with depression.

137   With regard to life events, depression occurs specifically following interpersonal loss compared with other mental disorders.

138   Life events are likely to be associated with the onset of depression.

139   Life events are qualitatively different in depressed patients compared with anxious patients.

140   With regard to life events, the risk of developing depression continues to increase with time after the event.

141   Autoscopy is essentially a primary delusion.

142   Autoscopy is a type of depersonalization experience.

143   Autoscopy is compatible with normality.

144   Autoscopy is a characteristic feature of right parietal/occipital infarct.

145   Autoscopy is the same as the doppelganger phenomenon.

146   Depersonalization is a normal human experience.

147   Hypnagogic hallucinations are normal human experiences.

148   Déjà vu is a normal human experience.

149   Irrational fear of harmless objects is a normal human experience.

150   Disorientation in time, place and person is a normal human experience.

151   Circumstantiality is a disorder of stream of thoughts.

152   Circumstantiality has been described as approximate answers in Ganser's syndrome.

153   Circumstantiality is synonymous with tangentiality.

154   Circumstantiality is a characteristic feature of schizophrenia.

155   Circumstantiality occurs in people with learning disability.

156   The terms 'pressure of speech' and 'flight of ideas' are interchangeable.

157   The terms 'blunted affect' and 'affective flattening' are interchangeable.

158   The terms 'dysphoria' and 'anhedonia' are interchangeable.

159   The terms 'made action' and 'delusion of control' are interchangeable.

160   The terms 'perseveration' and 'confabulation' are interchangeable.

[answers on page 165]

Dynamic psychopathology

161   Projective identification is equivalent to empathy.

162   Projective identification is the same as the ego defence mechanism of projection.

163   Projective identification is a characteristic ego defence mechanism associated with paranoid–schizoid position.

164   Projective identification is a primitive ego defence mechanism.

165   Projective identification is opposite to the ego defence mechanism of countertransference.

166   Ego strength is an important prerequisite for psychoanalytic therapy.

167   Ego strength is found to be very high amongst highly successful people.

168   Ego strength includes integrated interpretations.

169   Ego strength is developed during the anal stage.

170   Ego strength includes an ability to replace reality with fantasy.

171   In psychoanalytic theory, ego functions include mediation between the id and the outside world.

172   In psychoanalytic theory, ego functions include resolution of sexual conflict.

173   In psychoanalytic theory, ego functions include reality testing.

174   In psychoanalytic theory, ego functions include defensive functions.

175   In psychoanalytic theory, ego functions include object relationships.

176   Postulated psychodynamic factors in the aetiology of anxiety disorders include homosexual libidinal drives.

177   Postulated psychodynamic factors in the aetiology of anxiety disorders include threatened emergence into consciousness of forbidden repressed psychic conflicts.

178   Postulated psychodynamic factors in the aetiology of anxiety disorders include fear of castration.

179   Postulated psychodynamic factors in the aetiology of anxiety disorders include response to external threat.

180   Postulated psychodynamic factors in the aetiology of anxiety disorders include breaking of affectionate bonds.

181   The 'transitional object' as described in dynamic psychopathology is replaced by a permanent object, as the child grows older.

182   The 'transitional object' as described in dynamic psychopathology was first described by Melanie Klein.

183   The 'transitional object' as described in dynamic psychopathology represents a substitute for the mother's breast.

184   The 'transitional object' as described in dynamic psychopathology is an important component of the oedipal stage of psychosexual development.

185   The 'transitional object' as described in dynamic psychopathology is usually a favourite toy.

186   According to Freud's analysis of dreams, condensation is the reduction of one image into its component parts.

187   The concept of psychic determinism is that all mental activities are meaningful and purposeful.

188   The concept of psychic determinism is that all mental activities are random, accidental and meaningless.

189   The id is the psychic representation of drives which are largely unconscious.

[answers on page 167]

Clinical theory and skills

Aetiology

190   Heightened awareness of bodily sensations is considered to be an aetiological factor in somatization disorder.

191   Childhood sexual abuse is considered to be an aetiological factor in somatization disorder.

192   History of family illness during childhood is considered to be an aetiological factor in somatization disorder.

193   Excessive anxious preoccupation with illness is considered to be an aetiological factor in somatization disorder.

194   Misinterpretations of normal sensations as evidence of illness are considered to be an aetiological factor in somatization disorder.

195   Physical symptoms with no obvious organic cause are most likely to be due to a conversion disorder.

196   The onset of agoraphobia is generally associated with a panic attack.

197   In people over 65, suicide is commonly associated with Alzheimer's disease.

198   In delirium, a definite cause can be found in the majority of patients.

199   The limbic hypothalamic pituitary adrenal complex is implicated in the aetiology of severe mood disorders.

200   Cortisol may contribute to the cognitive impairment found in mood disorders.

[answers on page 168]

Classification/diagnosis

201   The reliability of diagnosis of schizophrenia is high with use of Bleuler's criteria.

202   The reliability and validity of diagnosis of mental disorders improves with the use of operational criteria.

203   The reliability of diagnosis of psychotic disorders is high because the criteria are polythetic.

204   The reliability of diagnosis in mental disorders is high for histrionic personality disorder.

205   The reliability of diagnosis in mental disorders is high for antisocial personality disorder.

206   The salient features that differentiate ICD-10 schizophrenia from DSM-IV schizophrenia include a lack of classification for the course of schizophrenia in ICD-10.

207   The salient features that differentiate ICD-10 schizophrenia from DSM-IV schizophrenia include absence of subtype simple schizophrenia in ICD-10.

208   The salient features that differentiate ICD-10 schizophrenia from DSM-IV schizophrenia include a longer duration of psychotic symptoms required to diagnose schizophrenia in ICD-10.

209   The salient features that differentiate ICD-10 schizophrenia from DSM-IV schizophrenia include exclusion of Schneider's first rank symptoms in the diagnostic criteria in ICD-10.

210 The salient features that differentiate ICD-10 schizophrenia from DSM-IV schizophrenia include a specific duration for the presence of prodromal symptoms in ICD-10.

211 Prodromal symptoms of schizophrenia in the ICD-10 include loss of interest in work.

212 Prodromal symptoms of schizophrenia in the ICD-10 include generalized anxiety.

213 Prodromal symptoms of schizophrenia in the ICD-10 include marked depression.

214 Prodromal symptoms of schizophrenia in the ICD-10 include auditory hallucinations.

215 Prodromal symptoms of schizophrenia in the ICD-10 include poor personal hygiene.

[answers on page 168]

History taking/interviewing

216 Medical students' interviewing skills can be improved by giving a detailed handout.

217 Medical students' interviewing skills can be improved by watching someone experienced interviewing patients.

218 Medical students interviewing skills can be improved by using structured interview schedules.

219 Medical students' interviewing skills can be improved by video feedback.

220 If a patient believes that Scotland Yard is listening to her telephone conversations, the physician should agree with the patient to establish rapport.

221 If a patient believes that Scotland Yard is listening to her telephone conversations, the physician should listen without agreeing or disagreeing.

222 In the clinical examination, questions about parental divorce, early childhood experiences or childhood friendships are considered developmental milestones.

223 In the clinical examination, questions about parental divorce, early childhood experiences or childhood friendships are considered as social history.

224 In the clinical examination, questions about parental divorce, early childhood experiences or childhood friendships are considered a personal inventory.

225   Divorce after 15 years of marriage in a 40-year-old woman is an example of internal stress.

226   Disorganization in an 18-year-old college student who is away from home for the first time is an example of internal stress.

227   Disclosure of clinical information is increased by the considered use of silences on the part of the interviewer.

228   Giving the patient a paradoxical injunction increases disclosure of clinical information.

229   Commenting on the patient's affect increases disclosure of clinical information.

230   Reasons for failure to clarify the extent of mood disorder include the interviewer's difficulty in dealing with emotion.

231   Reasons for failure to clarify the extent of a mood disorder include a failure to adhere to a standardized rating scale.

232   Agitation is usually seen as motor restlessness.

233   Agitation is usually associated with increased arousal.

234   Agitation is unusual in mixed affective disorders.

235   It is appropriate to ask a patient who has initially denied a history of past medical illness: 'Have you ever received prescribed medication for any ailment over the years?'

236   When taking a psychosexual history during the initial interview with a severely depressed married patient, it is usual to enquire about masturbatory fantasies.

237   Fluent speech is found in patients with subcortico-motor dysphasia.

238   Fluent speech is found in patients with receptive dysphasia.

239   Assessment of patients with schizophrenia must take into account their cultural factors.

[answers on page 169]

Mental state examination

240   With regard to cognitive testing in the elderly, the CAMCOG is part of a larger battery of tests: Cambridge Mental Disorders of the Elderly Examination (CAMDEX).

241   With regard to cognitive testing in the elderly, the Mini-Mental State Examination is helpful in distinguishing dementia from pseudodementia.

242   With regard to cognitive testing in the elderly, an assessment of aphasia is essential.

243   With regard to cognitive testing in the elderly, cognitive deficits can be detected by the Minnesota Multiphasic Personality Inventory (MMPI).

244   With regard to cognitive testing in the elderly, the Hachinski Scale is used to diagnose multi-infarct dementia.

245   Components of extended cognitive state examination include evaluation of language functions.

246   Components of extended cognitive state examination include level of consciousness.

247   Components of extended cognitive state examination include an evaluation of dyspraxia.

248   Components of extended cognitive state examination include visuospatial and constructional difficulties.

249   Components of extended cognitive state examination include an evaluation for formal thought disorder.

[answers on page 169]

Physical/neurological examination

250   In cerebellar disease, the involuntary tremors usually occur at rest.

251   Parkinsonian tremors usually have a rate of 4–7 cycles per second.

252   Fasciculations usually indicate a disease of lower motor neurones.

253   The involuntary movements of tardive dyskinesia persist during sleep.

254   Meige's syndrome is the eponymous label for blepharospasm.

255   Forced thinking is suggestive of an aura of complex partial seizures.

256   Nausea is suggestive of an aura of complex partial seizures.

257   Vomiting is suggestive of an aura of complex partial seizures.

258   Abdominal pain is suggestive of an aura of complex partial seizures.

259   Delusional mood is suggestive of an aura of complex partial seizures.

260   Absent knee and ankle jerks are characteristic features of Alzheimer's disease.

[answers on page 170]

Answers and explanations

Basic sciences

Basic psychology

1   **True**   Selective attention refers to the mechanisms by which only a few of the stimuli that we perceive are further processed. Broadbent described three types of processing involved. In filtering, stimuli are selected on the basis of a distinctive physical feature.

2   **False**

3   **True**   In pigeonholing, a bias is applied while attending and a stimulus is selected with less perceptual evidence than would normally be needed.

4   **False**

5   **True**   In categorizing, attention is paid to features of a stimulus, which show that it belongs to a certain stimulus class.

6   **False**   The description given here is that of escape training.

7   **False**   This is called 'reward training'.

8   **False**   This is a description of 'avoidance training'.

9   **False**   Punitive training has not been described, although a similar experiment is conducted for learned helplessness.

10   **False**   Habitual training does not exist.

11   **True**

12   **False**

Behavioural psychology

13   **False**

14   **True**

15   **False**

16   **True**   Functional analysis is a detailed examination of the precise circumstances surrounding the problem behaviour. It does not include analysis of defence mechanisms and psychotic symptoms. However, it includes a list of possible reinforcers that maintain the behaviour.

17   **True**   Learning that occurs by observing others is called observational learning. It is a very important form of learning in infancy and childhood.

18   **True**   Modelling uses the principle of observational learning therapeutically. It is an effective treatment for phobias wherein a fearless approach to a phobic situation is useful in motivating the patients to attempt to confront their phobias.

19   **True**

20   **False**   Respondent learning is the same as classical conditioning.

21   **True**

22   **True**

23   **False**   It is not a punishment. It is related to escape and avoidance learning.

24   **True**

Neuropsychology

25   **True**
26   **False**   It is a test of temporal lobe function. Benton visual retention test is designed to assess visual perception, visual memory and visuo-constructive abilities.
27   **False**

Human development

28   **True**
29   **True**
30   **False**

Psychopharmacology

General principles

31   **True**
32   **True**
33   **True**
34   **True**
35   **True**
36   **True**
37   **True**
38   **False**   It is an anticonvulsant drug. It is used in the treatment of bipolar disorders.
39   **True**
40   **True**
41   **False**   It is attributed to nigrostriatal blockade.
42   **True**   It parallels patient's recovery.
43   **False**   It occurs in both patients and normal healthy volunteers.
44   **True**
45   **False**
46   **False**
47   **False**
48   **True**
49   **True**

Pharmacokinetics

50   **True**
51   **True**
52   **True**

Pharmacodynamics

53   **False**   Reuptake into the presynaptic nerve terminal is a major mechanism for the active termination of neurotransmitter effects.
54   **True**

55   **True**   These factors play a role, with reduced expression of messenger RNA for some receptors following long-term treatment with agonists.
56   **False**
57   **True**   This is manifested as a reduction in agonist response. Several processes underlie receptor adaptation.
58   **True**   Benzodiazepines enhance the responsiveness of the GABA receptors and the inhibitory effects of GABA.
59   **True**
60   **True**
61   **True**   An example is zopiclone.
62   **False**   It blocks the action on $GABA_A$ receptors.
63   **True**
64   **True**
65   **True**   Ritanserin has anxiolytic properties.
66   **True**
67   **True**   They are also found in the cortex and olfactory system.

Adverse drug reactions

68   **True**
69   **True**
70   **False**
71   **False**
72   **True**
73   **False**
74   **False**
75   **False**
76   **False**
77   **False**   Reversible inhibitors of MAO A (RIMA) do not cause the cheese reaction that have been reported for the older generation of MAO inhibitors and they do not have the same restrictions. However, it is prudent not to indulge excessively in tyramine-containing products.
78   **False**   Tolerance develops to both ataxic and muscle relaxant properties, as well as to anticonvulsant properties.
79   **False**   Tolerance develops rapidly, so benzodiazepines are of little use in long-term prophylaxis.
80   **True**
81   **True**
82   **False**   Tolerance to sedation is greater than to psychomotor or amnesic effects, which is also greater than that to anxiolytic effects.
83   **False**
84   **False**
85   **False**
86   **False**
87   **True**   A symptom peculiar to benzodiazepine withdrawal is a sensation of abnormal body sway. Of particular note are abnormal perceptions such as hyperacusis, paraesthesias, photophobia and hypersensitivity to touch and pain.

Psychopathology

Descriptive

88 **True**   In some cases, the obsessions may be so bizarre that they may be difficult to distinguish from psychotic states.

89 **True**   By definition, obsessions cannot be ego-alien.

90 **False**   Resistance is not invariable and is not necessary to diagnose obsessions.

91 **False**   Activities that are pleasurable are sought and are not intrusive.

92 **True**   In magical thinking, thoughts, words or actions assume power and the person believes that they can prevent events, e.g. a person may count numbers to ward off danger.

93 **True**   The predominant presentation is with auditory hallucinations.

94 **True**

95 **False**   One of the features that distinguishes alcoholic hallucinosis is the occurrence of hallucinations in the setting of clear consciousness. However, visual hallucinations are not prominent in alcoholic hallucinosis.

96 **False**   It can also occur with continued drinking at reduced levels.

97 **True**

98 **True**

99 **False**

100 **True**

101 **True**   A diagnosis of depression is made as long as the patient currently satisfies the criteria for depression. Obsessions can occur in depressed patients and depression occurs in those who suffer from obsessions. If the patient's symptomatology meets the diagnostic criteria of depression in the presence of alcohol dependence, depression should be diagnosed.

102 **True**

103 **True**

104 **True**

105 **True**

106 **True**   Grief may be prolonged in the situations described in the above questions. For example, if the patient has died from acquired immune deficiency syndrome (AIDS), it might be difficult to acknowledge it publicly.

107 **False**   Irritability is a common presentation.

108 **False**

109 **False**   Distractibility underlies the decreased attention span rather than any alteration of consciousness.

110 **True**   Occurrence of this symptom in the early part of an episode makes it a useful early warning sign.

111 **True**

112 **False**   Alexithymia is not a diagnosis. It has been found in individuals who have somatoform illnesses such as somatoform pain disorder.

113 **False**

114 **False**   Alexithymia refers to an inability or difficulty expressing or being aware of one's feelings or moods.

115 **False**

116 **False**   Apart from what has been defined in answer 114, there are a number of features seen in people with alexithymia. They include not being psychologically introspective or imaginative.

117 **False**

118 **False**

119 **False**

120 **False**   No single feature distinguishes mania from schizophrenia; the diagnosis is based on several symptoms occurring together.

121 **True**

122 **True**

123 **False**

124 **False**

125 **False**

126 **False**

127 **True**

128 **True**

129 **False**

130 **False**

131 **False**

132 **False**

133 **False**

134 **True**

135 **True**

136 **True**

137 **False**   The relationship between depression and interpersonal loss is not specific as such events precede other disorders as well.

138 **False**   The symptom pattern of depression does not appear to be strongly related to life events.

139 **False**   Such a relationship has not been found.

140 **False**   The risk of developing depression tends to fall off with time after the event.

141 **False**

142 **False**

143 **True**   It can occur with migraine or epilepsy.

144 **False**

145 **True**   Autoscopy is an experience where one's own body image is perceived as being projected in external visual space. It is also known as the 'Doppelganger phenomenon'.

146 **True**

147 **True**

148 **True**

149 **True**

150 **False**

151 **True**

152 **False**

153 **False**

154 **False**

155 **True**   In circumstantiality, thinking is slowed down by trivial details, but it is goal-directed, whereas in tangentiality, the goal is never reached as thinking goes off into another direction.

156 **False**   Pressure of speech refers to the amount of speech produced whereas in flight of ideas, the train of thought changes from one subject to another rapidly.

157 **True**

158 **False**   Dysphoria is an unpleasant mood, while anhedonia means an inability to enjoy.

159 **True**   'Made' action is a specific example of a delusion of control.

160 **False**   Perseveration means meaningless or pointless repetition of words, ideas or themes. Confabulation is a memory disorder related to amnesia involving the generation of fabricated accounts of events experienced or facts either deliberately or without conscious intent to compensate for memory loss.

Dynamic psychopathology

161 **False**

162 **False**

163 **True**

164 **False**

165 **True**   Projective identification is also a projective mechanism although it is not synonymous with projection. Split off parts of an internal object are projected into another person. Mainly bad inner objects and bad parts of the self are projected. The object is then thought of as being persecutory. It also allows making oneself understood by exerting pressure on another individual to experience feelings similar to one's own.

166 **True**

167 **False**

168 **True**

169 **False**

170 **True**   Ego strength refers to the capacity of an individual to effectively engage in analysis. It also includes an individual's ability to regress temporarily, to be able to observe intrapsychic process and to function responsibly in a relationship.

171 **True**

172 **False**

173 **True**

174 **True**

175 **True**   Some of the main functions of the ego derive from its being an agency that mediates between the instinctual drives and the outside world. The capacity to form relationships that are mutually satisfying is also an important function of the ego.

176 True
177 True
178 True
179 False
180 True   Bowlby considered this to be a source of persistent anxiety.
181 False
182 False   It was described by Winnicott.
183 True
184 False
185 True   Transitional objects form an important aspect of object relations theory which deals with the involvement of ego with reality. They help the child to gradually move towards the acceptance of objective reality.
186 False
187 True
188 False
189 True

Clinical theory and skills

Aetiology

190 True
191 False   No relation with childhood sexual abuse has been suggested.
192 True
193 True
194 True   In somatization disorder, the aetiological factors involve contributions from several modalities, e.g. perception, cognition, affect and learnt behaviour.
195 False
196 True
197 False
198 True
199 True
200 True

Classification/diagnosis

201 False   When ill-defined subjective judgements are needed to determine presence of symptoms such as ambivalence and autism, the reliability is low.
202 False   Operational criteria only improve the reliability of diagnosis.
203 False   In mental disorders, diagnosis is based on multiple symptoms (polythetic) rather than one pathognomonic symptom (monothetic), thus lowering the reliability of diagnosis.
204 False
205 True   The diagnosis at least according to criteria in modern classification systems is based on well-defined behaviours, hence its reliability.

206 **False**

207 **False**   A subtype classified in ICD-10.

208 **True**

209 **False**

210 **False**   Duration of prodrome is not specified in ICD-10. However, duration of 6 months is specified for actual symptoms in the DSM-IV.

211 **True**

212 **True**

213 **False**

214 **False**

215 **True**   The prodromal symptoms are those symptoms which may precede the onset of psychosis by weeks or months. They include loss of interest in work, social activities, personal appearance and hygiene, together with generalized anxiety, mild degrees of depression and preoccupation.

History taking/interviewing

216 **True**

217 **True**

218 **False**

219 **True**

220 **False**

221 **True**

222 **True**

223 **False**

224 **False**

225 **False**

226 **True**   Internal stress may occur in an individual who is faced with a normal developmental task.

227 **True**

228 **False**

229 **True**

230 **True**

231 **False**

232 **True**

233 **True**

234 **False**

235 **True**

236 **False**

237 **False**

238 **True**

239 **True**

Mental state examination

240 **True**

241 **False**   It discriminates well between delirium and dementia.

242 **False**

243 **False**   MMPI is the Minnesota Multiphasic Personality Inventory which is a personality test.

244 **True**

245 **True**

246 **True**

247 **True**

248 **True**

249 **False**   If, after a routine examination of the cognitive state, the presence of an organic cerebral disorder is suspected, an extended evaluation is necessary.

Physical/neurological examination

250 **False**   Tremors occur during activity.

251 **True**

252 **True**   However, they can occur normally during fatigue or anxiety.

253 **False**

254 **False**   It is a combination of blepherospasm and oromandibular dyskinesia.

255 **True**

256 **False**

257 **False**

258 **True**

259 **False**

260 **False**

PAPER 7 (EMIs)

Note: In EMIs each option may be used once, more than once or not at all.

Questions

1 ICD-10 diagnosis of personality disorders

A Anankastic personality disorder
B Anxious (avoidant) personality disorder
C Dependent personality disorder
D Dissocial personality disorder
E Emotionally unstable personality disorder
F Histrionic personality disorder
G Paranoid personality disorder
H Schizoid personality disorder

For each of the following vignettes choose one option which best describes the vignette.

1   A 38-year-old single man lives with his parents. He is physically fit. His friends call him 'Mummy's boy' as he would ask his mother for almost everything. He finds it hard to live on his own when his parents go on holiday.

2   A 35-year-old single, unemployed man living alone. On several occasions, he has lost his temper, hurled abuse at the staff and customers in the supermarket. He has been charged with assaulting a staff member on one occasion. He says that he is unable to control himself when angry. He rationalizes his behaviour by saying that other people were rude to him. He often gets drunk and picks fights.

3   A 22-year-old single woman is admitted to the accident and emergency department after an overdose following an argument with her boyfriend. This is her sixth attendance in the last 4 months; each time has been after she took an overdose. She mentions that she has been prone to mood swings since she was a teenager. She also drinks in binges and has low self-esteem.

[answers on page 221]

2 Differential diagnosis of personality disorders

A Antisocial personality disorder
B Avoidant personality disorder
C Borderline personality disorder
D Delusional disorder
E Dependent personality disorder
F Narcissistic personality disorder
G Schizophrenia
H Schizotypal personality disorder

For each case history described below, choose the most appropriate diagnosis from the options above.

1   A 30-year-old single researcher is indignant when his college thesis panel refuses to approve his project. He says, 'They are jealous of me because they know I will be the most brilliant scientist in modern times'. He has had this type of attitude most of his life.

2   A 40-year-old single woman complains of being 'depressed since birth'. She lives with her elderly mother. She has low self-esteem. She believes that her mood has made it difficult for her to form relationships with men, for fear of being rejected. She has low self-esteem.

3   A 35-year-old single, unemployed woman lives alone. She becomes uncomfortable whilst queuing in the supermarket. She has lost her temper on several occasions, and hurled abuse at staff and customers at the supermarket. She has been charged with assaulting one of the staff at the checkouts. She says that she is unable to control her overwhelming urge to hit out when she has to wait.

[answers on page 221]

3 Differential diagnosis of catatonic signs

A Advertence
B Ambitendency
C Automatic obedience
D Catalepsy
E Cataplexy
F Echopraxia
G Mitgehen
H Posturing
I Waxy flexibility

Select one answer from the option list above for the following clinical situations.

1   A 49-year-old single man with a 10-year history of schizophrenia attended the
    clinic for a psychiatric review. When he was expected to shake his psychiatrist's
    hand, he initially put out his hand, then withdrew it, then extended it. He
    repeated this 10 times in rapid succession. His hand finally came to rest without
    touching the psychiatrist's hand.

2   A 27-year-old single woman suffers from paranoid schizophrenia. She takes her
    oral atypical antipsychotic drug regularly. She attends the outpatient clinic for
    a 6-month review. When the psychiatrist touched the back of her forearm with
    his index finger, her arm moved up. On continued touching, her upper arm
    stayed at shoulder level with the forearm flexed at the elbow.

3   A 38-year-old single man has been suffering from schizophrenia for several
    years. His mental state has been stable on antipsychotic medication. He attends
    the clinic for his 6-monthly review. The psychiatrist instructs him to raise his
    right arm. He raises both arms and stands up with the arms still raised. He
    repeated the movements every time he is asked to raise his right arm.

[answers on page 221]

4 Identification of the causes of mental disorders

A Acute intermittent porphyria
B Gasoline inhalation
C Hypothyroidism
D Hypoxia
E Lead poisoning
F Manganese intoxication
G Multiple sclerosis
H Premenstrual syndrome
I Vitamin B_{12} deficiency
J Wilson's disease (hepatolenticular degeneration)

For each of the following vignettes, choose one option which best describes the vignette.

1   A 45-year-old divorced man was found in a semiconscious state in his garage. His car engine was running and all the doors to the garage were closed. On clinical examination, he was confused and disorientated in time, place and person.

2   A 65-year-old woman has gradually become apathetic and moody. At times, she is confused and forgetful. She complains of tingling in her legs. On examination, her gait is unsteady and the deep tendon reflexes are exaggerated.

3   A 30-year-old married woman presents with a history of episodic anxiety, emotional liability, confusion and abdominal pain. She takes oral contraceptive pills but uses no other drugs.

[answers on page 221]

5 Identification of ego defence mechanisms

A Denial
B Displacement
C Isolation
D Magical undoing
E Projection
F Reaction formation
G Regression
H Repression

For each of the following vignettes, choose one option that will assist in establishing the defence mechanisms involved.

1   A 46-year-old woman who recently had an extramarital affair feels that her GP disapproves strongly of her behaviour. She believes that her behaviour was not really objectionable.

2   A 30-year-old woman who lost her husband suddenly after a massive myocardial infarction behaves as if there were nothing wrong. She continues to attend to daily chores and keeps talking about him as if he were still alive.

3   A 38-year-old woman is visiting her mother in a psychiatric inpatient unit. Her mother, aged 65 and who had been living alone, was admitted to the unit 2 weeks ago. She was found to be living in squalor and has been diagnosed as having dementia. Although the mother is well cared for by the staff on the unit, the daughter finds fault with everything that is done for her mother.

[answers on page 221]

6 Identification of signs and symptoms in acute confusional states

A Abdominal pain
B Ataxia
C Babinski's sign
D Flapping tremor
E Jaundice
F Nystagmus
G Ophthalmoplegia
H Petechial rash
I Pyrexia

For each of the following case scenarios, choose the most appropriate options that will assist in establishing the diagnosis. Follow the instruction given after each question.

1   A 27-year-old man is admitted to the medical ward with fever and vomiting. He is hepatitis B positive and has a history of alcohol dependence. On examination, he has an enlarged liver. (Choose the three best options.)

2   A 22-year-old female intravenous drug user is admitted to the medical ward. She is delirious and disorientated. (Choose the three best options.)

3   A 45-year-old man was found wandering in the street. He is disorientated in time, place and person and has a history of alcohol dependence for over 10 years. (Choose the three best options.)

[answers on page 221]

7 Investigations in patients suffering from acute and chronic confusional states

A Arterial blood gas
B Blood alcohol level
C Blood glucose
D Discussion with informant
E Liver function tests
F Mini-Mental State Examination
G Serum B_{12} levels
H Serum folate levels
I Skull radiograph
J Urea and electrolytes
K Urine drug screen

For each of the following case scenarios, choose the most appropriate options that will assist in establishing the diagnosis. Follow the instruction given after each question.

1   An 86-year-old male patient with a history of diabetes mellitus was admitted to the medical ward. He is confused and disorientated in time, place and person. He is mildly febrile. (Choose the three most appropriate investigations.)

2   A 22-year-old intravenous drug user was brought to the accident and emergency department after he tried to hang himself. He appears a little disorientated and disinhibited. His girlfriend informs the doctor that he was fine until 2 days ago. (Choose the three most appropriate investigations.)

3   A 44-year-old man with a long history of alcohol dependence is seen in the outpatient clinic. He has been increasingly forgetful. He also has some difficulties with walking due to an unsteady gait. (Choose the three most appropriate investigations.)

[answers on page 222]

8 Differential diagnosis of anxiety disorders

A Adjustment disorder
B Agoraphobia
C Generalized anxiety disorder
D Major depression
E Obsessive–compulsive disorder
F Panic disorder
G Post-traumatic stress disorder
H Social anxiety disorder (social phobia)

For each of the following vignettes, choose one option which best describes the vignette.

1 A 29-year-old single man presents to his general practitioner with a 2-year history of difficulties at work. His job requires him to make presentations to his colleagues and customers. He also reports that he has not visited the local pubs or restaurants recently, as he is worried that his behaviour may be embarrassing.

2 A 39-year-old married woman attends the accident and emergency department with three episodes of palpitations, sweating, hot flushes, trembling, choking sensation, fear of dying and churning in the stomach. These symptoms started about 2 months ago and they come suddenly without any warning.

3 A 46-year-old married man attends his general practitioner with a long history of repetitive and unpleasant thoughts. He believes that these thoughts are his own, but is unable to fight them off.

[answers on page 222]

9 Phenomenology of mental disorders

A Clang association
B Extracampine hallucination
C Haptic hallucinations
D Hygric hallucinations
E Hypnagogic hallucinations
F Pathological jealousy
G Pseudohallucinations
H Reflex hallucinations
I Vorbeireden
J Witzelsucht

For each of the descriptions given below, select one answer from the options list which describes it best.

1 A 21-year-old single unemployed man has been abusing cocaine and alcohol for a long time. He is quite sober and is fully oriented in time, place and person. However, he complains of feeling insects crawling under his skin. He is convinced that his body has been infested with lice in spite of no abnormal findings on physical examination and investigations.

2 A 45-year-old married man with no previous psychiatric history suffers from frontal lobe damage and becomes euphoric, with a tendency to joke and pun, making facetious remarks and indulging in silly pranks. There is no grandiosity or sleep disturbance or increased energy.

3 A 24-year-old single woman has been suffering from a chronic psychotic disorder for a few years. Her compliance with medication is good and she attends her outpatient appointments regularly. Her mental state is stable but she describes seeing God only when the bathroom tap is turned on.

[answers on page 222]

10 Differential diagnosis of acute and chronic confusional states

A Alcoholic dementia
B Alzheimer's disease
C Chronic subdural haematoma
D Delirium
E Frontotemporal dementia
F Multi-infarct dementia
G Normal pressure hydrocephalus
H Pick's disease

For each of the following vignettes, choose one option which best describes the vignette.

1   An 82-year-old previously healthy man was brought to the accident and emergency department by his wife. He appears malnourished and unkempt. It is evident that he has a significant but mild cognitive impairment. His wife gives a history of a fall about 2 months ago.

2   A 65-year-old single man attends the outpatient clinic with his brother for a psychiatric assessment. He gives a history of urinary incontinence, unsteady gait and mild cognitive impairment over several months.

3   An 84-year-old widow living alone is brought to the accident and emergency department by her neighbours. She was found wandering in the street last night. On examination, she is alert, but disoriented in time and place. The brain computed tomography scan shows some periventricular areas of radiolucency.

[answers on page 222]

11 Psychiatric diagnosis in elderly people

A Alcohol withdrawal syndrome
B Alzheimer's disease
C Charles Bonnet syndrome
D Cotard's syndrome
E Depression
F Generalized anxiety disorder
G Late-onset schizophrenia
H Obsessive–compulsive disorder
I Reduplicative paramnesia

For each of the following case histories, choose the most appropriate option.

1 A 72-year-old previously healthy woman develops a cataract over a period of time. She is functioning quite well. However, over the past few months she describes seeing blue dogs in the corner of her front room.

2 A 70-year-old married executive is admitted to the hospital for routine surgery. After about 48 hours in hospital and still not operated upon, he becomes acutely confused, anxious and agitated. He experiences prominent and frightening visual illusions.

3 An 89-year-old widower has become increasingly worried over the last 3 months, especially in the mornings. He has lost his confidence and his energy is low. His wife died about 6 months ago.

[answers on page 222]

12 Differential diagnosis of dementia

A Alcohol-related dementia
B Alzheimer's disease
C Binswanger's disease
D Dementia with Lewy bodies
E Frontal lobe dementia
F Huntington's disease
G Multi-infarct dementia
H Parkinson's disease

Choose one answer from the options list for each of the following vignettes. Each may be used once, more than once or not at all.

1 A 75-year-old man presents with significant memory loss for the past year. His family say that he has been seeing children playing in the living room for the past few months.

2 A 75-year-old man presents with a clinical picture suggestive of dementia. The neuropsychological tests show that he has relative preservation of memory but he has particular difficulties in the Trail Making Test and the Wisconsin Card Sorting Test.

3 A 45-year-old man presents to the outpatient clinic with his wife. He gives a 10-year history of bilateral involuntary choreiform movements. His wife has noticed gradual deterioration in his global cognitive functions over the last 2 years.

[answers on page 222]

13 Diagnosis of motor disorders in psychiatric patients

A Akathisia
B Catalepsy
C Cataplexy
D Chorea
E Dystonia
F Echopraxia
G Negativism
H Stereotypies
I Tardive dyskinesia
J Tics

For each of the following vignettes, choose one option which best describes the vignette.

1 A 65-year-old woman with a long history of bipolar affective disorder presents to the outpatient clinic for a review. Her husband says that her mental state has been stable for the past 5 years on an antipsychotic depot injection and antimanic (mood stabilizer) drug. However, over the past year he has noticed that she makes faces and grimaces at him and other members of the family.

2 A 45-year-old married woman presents to the accident and emergency department. She gives a history of recurrent falls to the ground, often following excitement or laughter.

3 A 20-year-old man was recently diagnosed as suffering from schizophrenia by his general practitioner. He was prescribed haloperidol in therapeutic doses about 5 days ago. He presents to the accident and emergency department with acute and distressing stiffness and rigidity of his neck since yesterday.

[answers on page 222]

14 Differential diagnosis of the patients presenting with confusion

A Alcohol withdrawal
B Alzheimer's disease
C Complex partial seizures
D Depression
E Hepatic encephalopathy
F Multi-infarct dementia
G Pneumonia
H Schizophrenia
I Subdural haematoma
J Wernicke's encephalopathy

For each of the following case scenarios, choose the most appropriate option.

1   An 80-year-old widower presents to the outpatient clinic with complaints of memory loss, difficulty in concentrating, loss of drive and interest over the past few months. His wife died 6 months ago. Physical examination reveals no apparent abnormality except weight loss. He scores 24 on the Mini-Mental State Examination.

2   A 45-year-old single woman is brought to the accident and emergency department by her friends with a history of acting strangely for 2 days. She stopped her usual treatment about two weeks ago. Her only complaint is an unpleasant taste in her mouth and a strange smell in the room. Her friends described her 'living in a world of her own'. On examination, she appeared preoccupied, perplexed and was disoriented in time and place. She has no fever or tremors.

3   A 70-year-old man with a history of hypertension and living alone has been in a state of neglect. His compliance with medication has been poor. He has difficulties with using his cooker and washing machine. At interview, he had his shirt poorly buttoned and his jumper was inside out. He was irritable and had word-finding difficulty.

[answers on page 223]

15 Causes of dementia

A Alzheimer's disease
B Cerebellar degeneration
C Frontal lobe dementia
D Gerstmann–Sträussler syndrome
E Huntington's disease
F Lewy body disease
G Multi-infarct dementia
H Normal pressure hydrocephalus
I Parkinson's disease

Select one answer from the options list for each of the following case scenarios.

1   A 70-year-old woman was found wandering at night. She was brought to the
     accident and emergency department. On examination, she was alert, but unable
     to give her address and telephone number or name the day and date. However
     she was able to give her full name, date of birth and names of her children. On
     physical examination all findings were normal.

2   A 76-year-old man has developed unsteady gait over several months. He has
     also become incontinent at times and is mildly disorientated in time, place and
     person. Lately, he has become forgetful.

3   A 63-year-old man is sent home on special leave from work because he had
     been making uncharacteristically rude remarks to younger female co-workers.
     He had also been cracking obscene jokes with strangers. His memory is relatively
     intact, but his word finding fluency is impaired.

[answers on page 223]

16 Causes of acute and chronic confusion

A Alcohol withdrawal syndrome
B Anticholinergic effects of tricyclic antidepressant drug
C Benzodiazepines
D Cerebral hypoxia
E Constipation
F Head injury
G Postoperative confusional state
H Transient ischaemia
I Urinary infection
J Water intoxication

For each of the following case scenarios, choose the single most likely cause of confusion from the options above.

1 A 45-year-old man was admitted following several falls 5 days ago. He has experienced periods of acute confusion since his admission. On examination, he has an enlarged liver, jaundice, coarse tremor and spider naevi. He is being treated with chlordiazepoxide and vitamin B complex.

2 A 75-year-old man has a transurethral resection of the prostate. On the second night after the operation, he becomes restless and confused. He is afebrile and the catheter urine is clear.

3 A previously healthy 90-year-old man had a repair of an inguinal hernia 5 days previously. He became incontinent and mildly confused over the last 2 days. A chest radiograph reveals normal findings.

[answers on page 223]

17 Causes of acute and chronic confusion

A Anticholinergic effects of an antipsychotic drug
B Cerebral hypoxia
C Communicating hydrocephalus
D Heart failure
E Hypoglycaemia
F Pneumonia
G Postoperative confusion
H Transient ischaemic attacks
I Vascular dementia
J Warfarin

For each of the following case scenarios, choose the single most likely cause of confusion from the options above.

1 A 75-year-old woman who is physically healthy was brought to the accident and emergency department by her family. She has been noticed to be mildly confused over the past week. Her mental state examination reveals paranoid delusions and visual hallucinations. She has been treated with a psychotropic drug by her general practitioner for the past 3 weeks.

2 A 78-year-old woman with a history of hypertension presents to the outpatient clinic with memory problems and transient focal neurological symptoms. She also gives a recent history of nocturnal confusion and stepwise deterioration in her mental health.

3 A previously well 82-year-old man wakes up during the middle of the night with slurred speech and unsteadiness. He is also reported to be mentally confused. He experienced some difficulties in finding his way to the toilet and putting on his clothes. He regained his full functions 4 hours later.

[answers on page 223]

18 Diagnosis of psychotic disorders

A Alcoholic hallucinosis
B Bipolar affective disorder
C Capgras' syndrome
D Late paraphrenia
E Othello syndrome
F Persistent delusional disorder
G Schizoaffective disorder
H Schizophrenia
I Schizophreniform disorder
J Schizotypal disorder

For each of the following vignettes, choose the one option which describes it best.

1   A 23-year-old single man is seen in the outpatient clinic. His family has noticed that he has been uninterested in his work for the past 2 years. He is socially withdrawn and has fallen out with his friends recently. He was seen to be laughing and giggling to himself on many occasions.

2   A 75-year-old partially deaf woman, who lives on her own, was admitted to the ward 3 days ago. She complains of some children entering her house and holding noisy parties every night and not leaving her alone. She is not amenable to any rational explanations.

3   A 34-year-old woman is seen in the outpatients' clinic. She believes that she is on a special mission to go to Rome and meet the Pope, to bring about peace on the earth. She has recently bought an expensive car without her husband's consent.

[answers on page 223]

19 Laboratory investigations to assist psychiatric diagnosis and management

A Arterial blood gases
B Cholesterol
C Creatinine clearance
D Creatinine kinase
E Erythrocyte sedimentation rate
F Full blood count
G Gamma glutamyl transferase
H Liver function test
I Serum prolactin level
J Thyroid function tests

For each of the following, choose the most appropriate laboratory test from the options above.

1 A 30-year-old man with schizophrenia was admitted to the psychiatric ward today. He has been receiving an antipsychotic depot injection and an oral antipsychotic drug for several months. He complained of muscular rigidity, elevated body temperature, weakness and thirst.

2 A 35-year-old woman with schizophrenia attends the outpatient clinic for her 6-monthly review. She mentions that she has been feeling well for a long time. However, she complains of weight gain, lack of libido and amenorrhoea of several months' duration. She would like to have a second child.

3 A 70-year-old previously healthy woman is referred to the outpatient clinic by her general practitioner. She was getting tired easily and had become sluggish in her reactions. She has also been feeling increasingly pessimistic for no apparent reason. She has experienced sleep disturbance over the past six months.

[answers on page 223]

20 Assessing suicidal intent/risk

A Beck's Depression Inventory
B Blood gases
C Discussion with informants
D Drug screen for analgesics
E Drug screen for narcotics
F Full blood count
G Liver function tests
H Mini-Mental State Examination
I Serum level of antimanic drug(s)
J Erythrocyte sedimentation rate

For each of the following case scenarios, choose the most appropriate options. Follow the instruction given after each question.

1   A 56-year-old man with a history of mood disorder was admitted to the medical ward following an overdose of some over-the-counter drugs. He gives a history of taking lithium for several years. On examination his physical condition is stable. He regrets his action and wants to be discharged home. (Choose the three best options.)

2   A 79-year-old widow living on her own was brought to the accident and emergency department by her son. She had been expressing suicidal thoughts for the past 2 weeks. She has been socially withdrawn, neglecting herself since her husband's death 6 months ago. She has been taking antihypertensive tablets for a long time. (Choose the two best options.)

3   A 48-year-old divorced man was admitted to the psychiatric ward a few days ago. He had made an attempt to take his life by hanging. He gives a history of depression and alcohol problems. On examination he is considered subjectively more depressed than on objective assessment. (Choose the three best options.)

[answers on page 223]

21 Physical examination of patients presenting with self-poisoning

A Ataxia
B Blurred vision
C Constricted pupils
D Dilated pupils
E Dysphagia
F Flapping tremors
G Labile blood pressure
H Hypotonia
I Nystagmus
J Normal respiration
K Sweating
L Tachycardia

For each of the following case scenarios, choose the most appropriate options. Follow the instruction given after each question.

1   A 17-year-old school leaver was brought to the accident and emergency department by his parents. He had gone to an all-night party with his mates the previous night. He has been abusing illicit drugs for the past 2 years. However, over the past 2 months he has been abusing amphetamines only as he liked the 'highs' he got with them. (Choose the three best options.)

2   A 19-year-old factory worker was brought to the accident and emergency department by his parents. After leaving school at 16, he had experimented with 'magic' mushrooms and other illicit drugs. However, later he enjoyed taking 'magic' mushrooms only. He tells the staff that he had a 'bad trip' last night. (Choose the three best options.)

3   A 23-year-old single, unemployed man was brought to the accident and emergency department by his family. He had been depressed for several months for no apparent reason. He started experimenting with illicit drugs 2 months ago. Over the past week he snorted substances containing phencyclidine. Last night he became belligerent, aggressive and untreatable. (Choose the three best options.)

[answers on page 224]

22 Physical examination of patients presenting with self-poisoning

A Bradycardia
B Cardiac arrhythmias
C Dilated reactive pupils
D Distended urinary bladder
E Dry skin
F Injected conjunctivae
G Pinpoint pupils unresponsive to light
H Postural hypotension
I Respiratory depression
J Seizures
K Tachycardia
L Vomiting and diarrhoea

For each of the following case scenarios, select the number of options according to the instructions.

1   A 56-year-old man with a long history of bipolar affective disorder was stabilized on lithium carbonate for several years. He became severely depressed following the unexpected sudden death of his wife 3 months ago. He was admitted to the medical ward following a serious overdose of his medication 8 hours ago. (Choose the two best options.)

2   A 71-year-old man with a history of benign prostatic hypertrophy became severely depressed 4 weeks ago. His general practitioner prescribed amitriptyline in therapeutic doses. He became suicidal over the past 5 days and took an overdose of his medication last night. He was brought to the accident and emergency department. (Choose the three best options.)

3   A 21-year-old single, unemployed man was brought to the accident and emergency department. He had gone to an all-night rave party with his friends. He had never taken any illicit drugs in the past. He tells the doctor that he had a 'bad trip' on cannabis which he had consumed for the first time. (Choose the three best options.)

[answers on page 224]

23 Physical examination of patients presenting with self-poisoning

A Blurred vision
B Broad-based gait
C Conjunctival injection
D Dilated reactive pupils
E Dry mouth
F Hypertension
G In-coordination
H Nystagmus
I Normal respiration
J Sweating
K Tremors
L Unsteady gait

For each of the following case scenarios, choose the most appropriate options. Follow the instruction given after each question.

1 A 36-year-old single city stock broker was brought to the accident and emergency department by his partner. He was under a lot of pressure at work over the past year. He took an overdose of cocaine, which he had been taking for the past 6 months. On examination, he is euphoric, but nervous and angry with the staff. (Choose the three best options.)

2 A 46-year-old housewife was admitted to the medical ward last night following an overdose of diazepam, which she had been taking for several years. She has been very worried about her daughter's forthcoming wedding which has caused her endless problems. (Choose the three best options.)

3 A 34-year-old divorced, unemployed man has been abusing alcohol for several years. Recently, he was evicted from his flat by the local authority and received a driving ban for drink driving offences. He consumed an excessive quantity of alcohol and tried to jump in front of the oncoming traffic last night. He was brought to the accident and emergency department. (Choose the three best options.)

[answers on page 224]

24 Managing suicidal risk in the accident and emergency department

A Admission to the psychiatric ward
B Compulsory admission under the Mental Health Act
C Discussion with an approved social worker
D Discussion with carers/family
E Outpatient follow-up
F Referral to clinical psychologist
G Referral to community mental health team (CMHT)
H Referral to general practitioner for follow-up
I Referral to medical team for admission
J Referral to surgical team

For each of the following case scenarios, choose the most appropriate initial course of action from the options above.

1   A 25-year-old woman attends the accident and emergency department with fresh superficial lacerations over both wrists, which do not require suturing. She is distressed and regrets her action. She has a number of old scars on both extremities. She had attended for similar reasons on a number of occasions over the past year.

2   A 19-year-old single woman is brought to the accident and emergency department following an overdose of 18 paracetamol tablets and alcohol. She had had a row with her boyfriend. She has no previous history of a mental disorder.

3   A 80-year-old widower, living on his own was brought to the accident and emergency department by his neighbours. He has been depressed since his wife's death 6 months ago. He has lost over a stone in weight. He does not want to live any longer without his wife. He refuses further help.

[answers on page 224]

25 Managing suicidal risk in the accident and emergency department

A Admission to a psychiatric ward
B Compulsory admission under the Mental Health Act
C Discussion with an approved social worker
D Outpatient follow-up
E Referral to drug and alcohol team
F Referral to general practitioner for further follow-up
G Referral to housing department
H Referral to medical team
I Referral to psychology service
J Referral to Samaritans

For each of the following case scenarios, choose the most appropriate initial course of action from the options above.

1   A 49-year-old man with severe alcohol problems for the past 20 years presents to the accident and emergency department. He had taken an overdose of diazepam with alcohol 4 hours previously. He is alert and requests help to get rid of his problems. He has never attended the hospital before. However, he has experienced visual hallucinations and shakes over the past week.

2   A 20-year-old man is brought to the accident and emergency department by his parents. He was noticed to be acting strangely over the past 3 days. He admits to taking illicit drugs. He is offered admission to the hospital but he is reluctant. His parents are not willing to take responsibility for him.

3   A 25-year-old single woman presents to the accident and emergency department following an overdose of 10 paracetamol tablets with alcohol following a row with her partner. She denies being suicidal any more and regrets her overdose which she took to teach her boyfriend a lesson. She wants to be discharged as soon as possible.

[answers on page 224]

26 Significant history in confirming a psychiatric diagnosis in deliberate self-harm

A Command auditory hallucinations
B History of a serious suicidal attempt
C Ideas of worthlessness and hopelessness
D Increased libido
E Multiple short-lived relationships
F Past history of violence and criminality
G Persecutory delusions
H Social isolation
I Substance misuse
J Unacceptable side effects of prescribed medication

For each of the following vignettes, choose the most important feature from options listed above to confirm the diagnosis.

1   A 25-year-old woman attends the accident and emergency department with multiple superficial lacerations on her wrists. She gives a history of repeated deliberate self-harm, homelessness and being intermittently employed over the past 5 years. She is diagnosed as having antisocial personality disorder.

2   A 23-year-old university graduate is brought to the accident and emergency department by her partner, having been prevented from jumping out of the first floor window. She believed that she could fly and had special powers to rid the world of poverty. She is considered to be in a hypomanic state.

3   A 20-year-old woman is brought to the accident and emergency department following an overdose of 10 paracetamol tablets. She had dropped out of her university course. She had become socially withdrawn over the past year. She is convinced that she is being followed by some unknown people. She is considered to be suffering from schizophrenia.

[answers on page 224]

27 Significant history in confirming a psychiatric diagnosis in deliberate self-harm

A Anhedonia
B Distorted body image
C Early morning waking
D History of serious suicidal attempt
E Loss of appetite
F Overactivity
G Persecutory delusions
H Social isolation
I Transient psychotic symptoms
J Weight loss

For each of the following vignettes, choose the most important feature from options listed above to confirm the diagnosis.

1   A 26-year-old single woman is referred to the outpatient clinic with a 5-year history of severe dieting. She had been exercising regularly and taking regular purgatives to stay slim. Her body mass index is 12. She does not want to live any longer. A diagnosis of anorexia nervosa is considered.

2   A 41-year-old man who is separated from his wife was brought to the accident and emergency department following an attempt to take his life by joining a hose-pipe to the car exhaust. He had been fed up and depressed since his wife left him 6 months ago. A diagnosis of depression is considered.

3   A 46-year-old divorced woman presents to the accident and emergency department following an overdose of 10 paracetamol tablets. She has a history of unaccountable acts of superficial deliberate self-harm over the past 5 years. She is irritable and gets angry for no apparent reason and tends to blame others for her problems. A diagnosis of borderline personality disorder is considered.

[answers on page 225]

28 Assessing suicidal risk

A Beck's Depression Inventory
B Creatinine clearance
C Discussion about suicidal intent
D Drug screen for alcohol
E Drug screen for amphetamines
F Drug screen for analgesics
G Drug screen for hallucinogens
H Hamilton Depression Rating Scale
I Montgomery–Asberg Depression Rating Scale
J Urea and electrolytes

For each of the following case scenarios, choose the most appropriate initial action from the options above, which will assist in completing the assessment.

1   A 57-year-old widower was brought to the accident and emergency department following an attempt to take his by life by hanging. He gives a history of depression and alcohol abuse since his wife's death a year ago. He also informs staff that he has not touched alcohol for over a week now. He regrets his action and wants to go home.

2   A 20-year-old woman was brought to the accident and emergency department following a night out at a local pub. Her behaviour is bizarre, unpredictable and disinhibited. Her mood is elated. She believes that she is a princess and can also fly like a bird.

3   A 27-year-old single woman was brought to the accident and emergency department following an overdose of painkillers with alcohol about 6 hours ago. She is conscious and cooperative during her interview but denies being suicidal any longer. She admits to being depressed since her boyfriend left her 3 months ago.

[answers on page 225]

29 Investigations in patients suffering from acute and chronic confusional states

A Blood culture
B Blood glucose
C Electroencephalogram
D Full blood count
E Liver function tests including gamma-glutamyl transferase
F Mid-stream urine culture
G Magnetic resonance imaging (MRI) scan
H Serum level of antimanic drug(s)
I Urea and electrolytes
J Urine drug screen

For each of the following case scenarios, choose the single most important option from the list above that will assist in establishing the diagnosis.

1   A 39-year-old man is brought to the accident and emergency department in an excitable, agitated and confused state. He has been abusing alcohol for a few years. He had stopped drinking 3 days ago. On examination, he is pyretic, tremulous with shakes and is trying to fight with people around him.

2   A 22-year-old woman is brought to the accident and emergency department in an excitable and confused state. She had been out last night with her friends to a local night club. She has no previous psychiatric history. On examination, she has dilated but reactive pupils, tachycardia and labile affect.

3   A 41-year-old woman was knocked over by a passing vehicle while she was crossing the road outside her house around 2 pm. She did not lose consciousness and continued with her household chores. When her husband came home from work around 6 pm, he found her mentally confused and brought her to the accident and emergency department.

[answers on page 225]

30 Investigations in patients suffering from acute and chronic confusional states

A Chromosomal analysis
B Computed tomography (CT) scan
C Differential blood count
D Echocardiogram
E Electrocardiogram
F History from the carers
G Mid-stream urine analysis
H Mid-stream urine culture
I Mini-Mental State Examination
J MRI scan

For each of the following case scenarios, choose the single most appropriate option.

1   An 80-year-old woman is admitted to the ward having been found wandering on the streets. She has no previous psychiatric history. On examination, she is pyrexial with tachycardia and tenderness over her lower abdomen. She has been incontinent over the past few days.

2   A 70-year-old woman is admitted to the ward as her husband was unable to cope with her. Over the past few years, she has become forgetful, cantankerous and socially withdrawn. At times she does not recognize her husband which he finds very distressing.

3   A 45-year-old married man is brought to the accident and emergency department by his wife. He has been suffering from involuntary bilateral choreiform movements for several years. More recently he has become forgetful and withdrawn. His physical examination reveals no other abnormalities.

[answers on page 225]

31 Differential diagnosis of psychotic disorders

A Alcohol hallucinosis
B Bipolar affective disorder
C Brief psychotic disorder
D Capgras' syndrome
E Othello syndrome
F Persistent delusional disorder
G Schizoaffective disorder
H Schizophrenia
I Schizophreniform disorder
J Schizotypal disorder

For each of the following vignettes, choose one option which best describes the vignette.

1 A 59-year-old spinster who lives alone believes that she was being monitored by Scotland Yard for the past 10 years, in spite of having done nothing wrong. She would not accept the possibility that she could be mistaken in her belief. She writes copious letters to the Queen complaining about her problems.

2 A 45-year-old separated man presents to the accident and emergency department complaining of accusatory and threatening voices without any explanation. He gives a 10-year history of excessive drinking. On examination he is alert, cooperative and fully orientated in time, place and person.

3 A 51-year-old married man visits his general practitioner complaining that his wife has been behaving in a strange and bizarre manner for the past 6 months. He also believes that she is not the same person he had known and in fact is someone else in disguised as his wife. The general practitioner who has met his wife several times disagrees with him and offers a referral to the psychiatrist for further assessment.

[answers on page 225]

32 Diagnosis of common mental disorders

A Agoraphobia
B Anorexia nervosa
C Bulimia nervosa
D Delirium
E Delirium tremens
F Panic disorder
G Phobic anxiety disorder
H Post-traumatic stress disorder
I Schizophrenia
J Social phobia

For each of the following vignettes, choose the most appropriate diagnostic category from the options list above.

1   A 20-year-old male student is brought to the outpatient clinic by his mother who is concerned about him. He was fine until 6 months ago. He has been noticed to be socially withdrawn and isolated. He lacks motivation in his study and spends a lot of time in his room talking to himself. He denies anything is wrong with him.

2   A 83-year-old woman is recovering from a hip replacement operation. She has become pyrexial, agitated and confused over the past 2 days. She is also restless and keeps pulling out her drip. On examination, she is able to give her name and date of birth but not the day, date or month.

3   A 35-year-old single woman attends the outpatient clinic complaining of palpitations, tension, headaches, nervousness, feeling of choking, chest pains and trembling for several years. Her symptoms usually appear when she goes for a drink or dinner with her friends.

[answers on page 225]

33 Identification of signs and symptoms in a mental state examination

A Auditory hallucinations
B Impaired concentration
C Depressed mood
D Flight of ideas
E Illusion
F Disorientation in time, place and person
G Paranoid delusions
H Pressure of speech
I Thought blocking
J Thought broadcasting

For each of the following vignettes, choose the option that best matches the description of the vignette.

1 A 41-year-old man attends the accident and emergency department along with his spouse. During the conversation he says, 'How are you doctor? I come from Birmingham and live in London. Where did you get that tie? It looks like it's left over from the sixties. I like the warm weather of Australia. Is that photograph of your wife? Have you ever been on holiday to America?'

2 A 74-year-old man is brought to the outpatient clinic by his wife. He has not spoken to other people for the past few weeks. On examination he appears dishevelled and unkempt. He is mute and keeps looking at the floor, with drawn angles of his mouth.

3 A 21-year-old man, previously healthy, is brought to the accident and emergency department by his mother. He had experimented recently with illicit drugs. He believes that he is hunted by a terrorist organization since his recent visit to Israel.

[answers on page 226]

34 Identification of signs and symptoms in a mental state examination

A Audible thoughts
B Blunted affect
C Inappropriate affect
D Insight
E Judgement
F Obsessional ruminations
G Tangentiality
H Thought blocking
I Thought withdrawal
J Visual hallucinations

For each of the following vignettes, choose the option that best matches the description of the vignette.

1   A 27-year-old man was admitted to the ward 3 days ago. He has no previous psychiatric history. He believes that his thoughts are no longer private as the staff and patients receive them from the television.

2   A 25-year-old single woman presents herself to the accident and emergency department as she has been very upset since her boyfriend left her 3 days ago. She admits to being suicidal but claims that she would not carry it out. She requests to see a psychiatrist.

3   A 19-year-old student presents to the accident and emergency department following a night out with his friends to a local night club. He looks perplexed and anxious. During the conversation he pauses intermittently for a few minutes and says that he keeps losing his chain of thought.

[answers on page 226]

35 Application of patient interviewing techniques

A Clarification
B Confrontation
C Direct question
D Expressing empathy
E Interpretation
F Open-ended question
G Recapitulation
H Suggestion

For each of the scenarios described below, choose the SINGLE most appropriate option that it best exemplifies.

1   A 30-year-old single man presents himself to the accident and emergency department following an overdose. The examining doctor starts the interview by asking, 'How are you feeling now?'

2   A 19-year-old woman attends the accident and emergency department following a fight with her boyfriend. She is in severe pain. The examining doctor asks her, 'Where is your pain located?'

3   A 35-year-old man attends the outpatient clinic following a fall at work. The examining doctor asks the patient, 'You say that you back pain occurs only at work. Tell me more about the nature of your work.'

[answers on page 226]

36 Application of patient interviewing techniques

A Clarification
B Closed question
C Confrontation
D Expressing empathy
E Facilitation
F Interpretation
G Open-ended question
H Reflection

For each of the scenarios described below, choose the SINGLE most appropriate option that it best exemplifies.

1   A 45-year-old divorced man attends the outpatient clinic for a review of his condition. He has a serious problem with excessive drinking. During the interview the doctor tells the patient, 'You plan to continue drinking in spite of my advice to remain completely abstinent.'

2   A 32-year-old woman attends the outpatient for a medico-legal report following a road traffic accident. The examining doctor says to her, 'You seem very angry with the driver of the third party vehicle involved in the accident. I wonder if you blame him for what happened.'

3   A 75-year-old man is brought to the accident and emergency department by his daughter. He had been depressed since his wife died 3 months ago. The examining doctor asks the patient, 'You said your symptoms began after your wife's death?'

[answers on page 226]

37 Application of patient interviewing techniques

A Clarification
B Closed question
C Expressing empathy
D Facilitation
E Interpretation
F Open-ended question
G Suggestion
H Summarization

For each of the scenarios described below, choose the SINGLE most appropriate option that it best exemplifies.

1   A 29-year-old man who has been depressed for 6 months attends the outpatient clinic. He has an acrimonious relationship with his father who wants him to stand on his own two feet. During the interview, the examining doctor remarks, 'You seem to be very angry and annoyed about your illness. Perhaps you feel that your father is responsible for it.'

2   A 21-year-old student is brought to the accident and emergency department following a fight with some strangers. He had a lot to drink during the night. He is alert and fully conscious and complains of being uncomfortable with abdominal pain. The examining doctor remarks, 'You must be feeling a lot of pain at the moment.'

3   A 76-year-old woman attends the outpatient clinic for assessment of her depression. She became unwell following her husband's death 4 weeks ago. During the interview the examining doctor remarks, 'You must be feeling terrible and your life must have turned upside down since your husband's death.'

[answers on page 226]

38 Application of patient interviewing techniques

A Clarification
B Closed question
C Confrontation
D Expressing empathy
E Facilitation
F Interpretation
G Recapitulation
H Reflection

For each of the scenarios described below, choose the SINGLE most appropriate option that it best exemplifies.

1   A 61-year-old retired woman attends the outpatient clinic. She has no previous psychiatric history. After initial introductions the examining doctor asks her, 'What would you like me to help you with?'

2   A 39-year-old man presents to the accident and emergency department. He has been feeling very low since his wife left him without any warning 6 weeks ago. He has not been coping with his two children who live with him. During the interview, the examining doctor remarks, 'You must be going through difficult times at present. I can understand how you are feeling.'

3   A 55-year-old woman attends the outpatient clinic for assessment of her anxiety disorder. At the end of the interview, the examining doctor says to her, 'Let me see if I have got it right, Your trouble started after the road traffic accident you had some 6 months ago. It is getting worse and you are still suffering.'

[answers on page 226]

39 Clinical applications of interviewing techniques

A Clarification
B Closed question
C Confrontation
D Empathy
E Interpretation
F Open-ended question
G Recapitulation

For each of the scenarios described below, choose the SINGLE most appropriate option that it best exemplifies.

1   During the consultation with his doctor, a 50-year-old man tries to describe his problems. However, the doctor finds him rather vague and asks, 'Where is your pain located? Can you point to it with only one finger?'

2   The consultation continues. After a while, the doctor says to him, 'You say your back pain occurs only at work. Tell me more about the nature of your work.'

3   The doctor tells his patient, 'You seem to be very angry and annoyed about your illness. Perhaps your father is responsible for it?'

[answers on page 226]

40 Differential diagnosis of psychosomatic syndromes

A Body dysmorphic disorder
B Chronic fatigue syndrome
C Conversion disorder
D Depression
E Generalized anxiety disorder
F Hypochondriasis
G Pain disorder
H Somatization disorder

For each of the following vignettes, choose the best option.

1   A 40-year-old married accountant is seen in the outpatient clinic with a 3-year history of extreme lethargy, poor sleep, vague aches and pains and headaches. He gives a history of recurrent sore throat prior to the onset of his symptoms. After periods of physical exertion, he often takes himself to bed for several days. Blood tests including liver functions, thyroid functions and blood glucose are within normal range.

2   A 39-year-old woman is admitted with multiple physical complaints including headaches, blurred vision, weakness, numbness, urinary frequency, intermittent diarrhoea, bloating and palpitations. Extensive physical investigations reveal normal findings.

3   A 26-year-old single man has seen several medical practitioners because he believes that he is infected with the human immunodeficiency virus (HIV) following a casual unprotected one night stand. He has had repeated blood tests which have all been negative. After each negative test he is temporarily reassured before he presents with renewed fears of HIV. He is not a drug user.

[answers on page 227]

41 Differential diagnosis of anxiety disorders

A Agoraphobia
B Claustrophobia
C Generalized anxiety disorder
D Major depression
E Mixed anxiety and depressive disorder
F Obsessive compulsive disorder
G Panic disorder
H Social phobia

For each of the following vignettes, choose the option that best matches the description of the vignette.

1   A 40-year-old married woman presents to the accident and emergency department. She was shopping in a supermarket for about half an hour before she suddenly experienced palpitations, breathlessness, dizziness, chest pains and fears that she was going to die. She says that these symptoms occur 4–6 times a month and are not related to any particular situation.

2   A 46-year-old married man presents to his general practitioner with complaints of tightness in chest, choking, difficulty in swallowing, palpitations, severe initial insomnia and inability to relax. His symptoms have gradually got worse since he was made redundant 5 months ago.

3   A 23-year-old postgraduate student in biological sciences presents to his general practitioner for a prescription of an anxiolytic drug. He informs the doctor that he feels very nervous and anxious about presenting his project next week fearing ridicule from his tutor and colleagues. He has managed similar situations in the past with great difficulty.

[answers on page 227]

42 Differential diagnosis of mood disorders

A Bipolar I disorder
B Bipolar II disorder
C Cyclothymic disorder
D Dysthymic disorder
E Generalized anxiety disorder
F Major depressive disorder, recurrent
G Mood disorder due to a general medical condition
H Schizoaffective disorder

For each of the following case scenarios, choose the option that describes it best.

1   A 49-year-old male accountant presents to his general practitioner with an 8-week history of worsening depression, early morning waking, weight loss, reduced libido, poor concentration, tiredness and suicidal thoughts. He believes that his evil thoughts had caused the recent death of his wife. He has had such episodes in the last 10 years.

2   A 52-year-old woman with no previous psychiatric history presents with a 6-month history of fatigue, loss of interest and energy, and poor concentration. Physical examination reveals no abnormality. Laboratory investigations reveal a thyroid stimulating hormone (TSH) level of 16.5.

3   A 42-year-old man presents with low mood, loss of interest, and irritability over the past two months. He has a past history of episodes of feeling over the moon, with little need for sleep and undue overactivity. These episodes would last for a few days at a time. While these episodes have been disruptive, he has so far avoided hospital admission.

[answers on page 227]

43 Mechanisms of adverse drug interactions

A Blockade of mesolimbic D_2 receptors
B Blockade of striatal D_2 receptors
C Discontinuation reaction
D Downregulation of serotonin receptors
E QT_C prolongation
F Stimulation of histaminic receptors
G Stimulation of 5-HT_3 receptors
H Stimulation of 5-HT_{1A} receptors
I Torsades de pointes

For each of the following clinical situations, choose the most appropriate options. Follow the instruction given after each question.

1 A 35-year-old depressed woman fails to respond to treatment with paroxetine 30 mg daily for 8 weeks. Paroxetine is stopped abruptly and the next day, she is commenced on dosulepin 75 mg nocte. Four days later, she attends her general practice complaining of nausea, headache, dizziness and paraesthesia. (Choose the two best options.)

2 A 60-year-old woman suffering from a severe and enduring mental illness has been treated with pimozide. She develops a severe throat infection and is treated with clarithromycin. Two days later she faints for no apparent reason. (Choose the two best options.)

3 A 30-year-old man suffering from bipolar affective disorder is treated with risperidone. He develops cog-wheel rigidity and a pill-rolling tremor. (Choose the single best option.)

[answers on page 227]

44 Identification of drug interactions

A Amiloride
B Carbamazepine
C Diazepam
D Enalapril
E Lidocaine
F Losartan potassium
G Modafinil
H Procyclidine
I   Sertindole
J Thioridazine
K Topiramate

For each of the following clinical situations, choose the most appropriate options. Follow the instruction given after each question.

1   A 50-year-old woman with bipolar affective disorder has been taking lithium carbonate for several years. She becomes drowsy, ataxic and complains of tinnitus. The serum lithium level is 2.2 mmol/L. (Choose the three best options.)

2   A 30-year-old woman becomes pregnant despite taking her oral contraceptive pill meticulously. (Choose the three best options.)

3   A 75-year-old man has been treated with fluoxetine 20 mg daily over the past 5 years. He becomes disorientated in time, place and person. He is drowsy. An electrocardiographic recording shows prolonged QT interval. (Choose the three best options.)

[answers on page 227]

45 Differential diagnosis of somatoform disorders

A Briquet's syndrome
B Concussion
C Conversion disorder
D Dissociative amnesia
E Fugue
F Korsakoff's syndrome
G Hypochondriasis
H Psychogenic pain disorder
I Retrograde amnesia

For each of the following clinical situations, choose the most appropriate options. Follow the instruction given after each question.

1 A 35-year-old previously healthy Gulf War soldier had returned home from his duties a few months ago. He has now been asked to rejoin his colleagues. He suddenly finds his right hand paralysed. (Choose the single best option.)

2 A 26-year-old man attends the accident and emergency department complaining of being hit on the head while crossing the road, which he claimed occurred 3 days earlier, in a town some 60 miles away. On further enquiry, he stated that he could not recall his name or address or how he arrived at the hospital. However, he was aware of the day and date. (Choose the two best options.)

3 A 35-year-old married woman consults her general practitioner complaining of abdominal pain, nausea and bloating. Her physical examination is normal, as is a subsequent range of investigations. The medical notes indicate that over the past 5 years, she had attended repeatedly with a wide range of complaints, including pain at various sites, menstrual disturbances and double vision. She has attended several specialists, who have not identified physical causes sufficient to explain her symptoms. (Choose the two best options.)

[answers on page 227]

46 Differential diagnosis of psychotic disorders

A Alcoholic hallucinosis
B Chronic amphetamine misuse
C Fahr's syndrome
D Huntington's disease
E Metachromatic disease
F Neurosarcoidosis
G Partial complex seizures
H Mental and behavioural disorder due to phencyclidine use

For each of the following clinical situations, choose one option from the list above.

1   A 39-year-old married man presents with persecutory delusions, depressive symptoms, aggressive behaviour, clumsiness and mild mental confusion. On examination, he has an unsteady gait and increased muscle tone. An electroencephalogram (EEG) shows poorly developed alpha rhythms and a positron emission tomography (PET) scan shows hypoperfusion of the caudate nucleus. He has no prior psychiatric history. His family history is unknown.

2   A 29-year-old single man recently arrived from North America, presents with paranoid delusions, thought disorder and outbursts of bizarre behaviour. He is socially withdrawn. He gives a recent history of seizures and periods of mild confusion. He was well until 2 months ago.

3   A 32-year-old woman presents with fluctuating psychotic and depressive symptoms and agitation. On examination, she has facial nerve palsy, nodular lesions on her legs and mild pyrexia. She has a history of respiratory problems.

[answers on page 227]

47 Risk factors for mental illness in older people

A Being a member of a minority ethnic group
B Currently single
C Deafness
D Female gender
E Hypertension
F Living alone
G Longer period of education
H Low levels of exercise
I Male gender
J Older age

For each of the following clinical situations choose the risk factor(s) from the options above for which there is an evidence base. Follow the instruction given after each question.

1 A 78-year-old retired doctor, whose wife died 6 months ago, has had a recent cerebrovascular accident. He recovered physically and has no cognitive impairment. However, he has recently begun to feel sad and hopeless and that life was not worth living. He refuses to eat and has interrupted sleep, which does not refresh him. (Choose the three best options.)

2 An 80-year-old widow with a 3-year history of Alzheimer's disease has recently become tearful with early morning wakening and weight loss. She has lost interest in attending the day centre. (Choose the two best options.)

3 A 66-year-old retired computer programmer recently developed a belief that he was being followed by the police. He also believes that the Prime Minister had told him that he did not have to pay council tax. He therefore stopped paying the tax about 6 months ago. He is in danger of being evicted from his supported living accommodation. (Choose the three best options.)

[answers on page 228]

48 Differential diagnosis of mental disorders presenting with physical symptoms

A Body dysmorphic disorder
B Briquet's syndrome
C Conversion disorder
D Delusional disorder
E Obsessive compulsive disorder
F Panic disorder
G Post-traumatic stress disorder
H Schizophrenia

For each of the following clinical situations, choose the most appropriate option(s). Follow the instruction given after the question.

1 A 29-year-old Nigerian woman presents with a 2-week history of being unable to speak, which began suddenly after witnessing an assault. On examination, she is able to mouth words but is unable to vocalize them. She is noted to cough audibly. She is alert and communicates well by writing. (Choose the single best option.)

2 The wife of a 27-year-old man is concerned that he has stopped speaking recently. He was discharged from the hospital 4 weeks earlier. On examination, he appears fearful, guarded and reluctant to raise his voice above a whisper. When left alone in the examination cubicle, he is observed to shake his head and make odd movements of his hands. (Choose the two best options.)

3 A 35-year-old woman takes up to 25 baths every day in an attempt to rid herself of what she describes as an unbearable infestation with lice. On examination, there was no evidence of such infestation. She was functioning well otherwise. (Choose the single best option.)

[answers on page 228]

49 Differential diagnosis of mood disorders

A Agoraphobia
B Bipolar affective disorder
C Borderline personality disorder
D Dysthymia
E Generalized anxiety disorder
F Major depression
G Panic disorder
H Schizophrenia

For each of the following clinical scenarios, choose one or more likely options(s). Follow the instruction given after the question.

1   A 21-year-old university student presents for the first time with a history of persecutory ideas, low mood, poor sleep, a sense of vagueness and perplexity. He denies hallucinations and thought interference. His maternal uncle suffers from a severe and enduring mental illness. He is currently unable to cope with his studies. (Choose the two best options.)

2   A 79-year-old widow complains of low mood, feeling miserable, with a sense of hopelessness and uselessness and recurrent suicidal thoughts. These symptoms have been getting progressively worse over the past 6 months. Her cognitive functions are intact except for poor attention and concentration. She sleeps well but her appetite is poor with significant recent weight loss. (Choose the single best option.)

3   A 34-year-old single woman who lives alone presents to the accident and emergency department following an overdose and self-inflicted superficial wound. She has had several boyfriends over the years but currently is not in any relationship. She shows considerable anger towards both the nursing and medical staff. She admits feeling depressed and suicidal almost continuously. (Choose the single best option.)

[answers on page 228]

50 Differential diagnosis of anxiety disorders

A Adjustment disorder
B Depressive disorder with somatic symptoms
C Episodic paroxysmal anxiety
D Generalized anxiety disorder
E Mixed anxiety and depressive disorder
F Panic disorder
G Social anxiety disorder (Social phobia)
H Somatization disorder

For each of the following vignettes, choose the option(s) which best describe(s) the vignette. Follow the instruction given after the question.

1 A 36-year-old man presents to his general practitioner with complaints of epigastric discomfort, chest pains, headaches, palpitations, dizziness, and jelly-like legs intermittently for several months. His wife, a passenger in his car, was killed in a road traffic accident a year ago. He often feels tearful, and it is worse when he travels by car. (Choose the two best options.)

2 A 37-year-old single woman feels anxious whenever she has to go out. She often wakes up feeling anxious on days when she knows she has to go out. Her anxiety gets worse throughout the morning until the time she has to leave the house. She feels faint and fears she might drop dead. She has frequently returned home without completing her shopping. (Choose the single best option.)

3 A 48-year-old married man complains of feeling anxious, poor appetite and weight loss. He has become socially withdrawn, and feels uncomfortable whilst visiting friends. Although he makes an effort to go out, he often returns home early. He has started drinking heavily, particularly when he has to meet his friends. (Choose the two best options.)

[answers on page 228]

Answers

1 ICD-10 diagnosis of personality disorders

1   C
2   D
3   E

2 Differential diagnosis of personality disorders

1   F
2   B
3   A

3 Differential diagnosis of catatonic signs

1   B
2   G
3   C

4 Identification of the causes of mental disorders

1   D
2   I
3   A

5 Identification of ego defence mechanisms

1   E
2   A
3   E

6 Identification of signs and symptoms in acute confusional states

1   A, D, E (Hepatic failure)
2   A, H, I (Bacterial septicaemia)
3   B, F, G (Wernicke's encephalopathy)

7 Investigations in patients suffering from acute and chronic confusional states

1   C, D, J
2   A, B, K
3   E, G, H

8 Differential diagnosis of anxiety disorders

1   H
2   F
3   E

9 Phenomenology of mental disorders

1   C
2   J
3   H

10 Differential diagnosis of acute and chronic confusional states

1   C
2   G
3   B

11 Psychiatric diagnosis in the elderly

1   C
2   A
3   E

12 Differential diagnosis of dementia

1   D
2   E
3   F

13 Diagnosis of motor disorders in psychiatric patients

1   I
2   C
3   E

14 Differential diagnosis of the patients presenting with confusion

1   D
2   C
3   F

15 Causes of dementia

1   A
2   H
3   C

16 Causes of acute and chronic confusion

1   A
2   D
3   I

17 Causes of acute and chronic confusion

1   A
2   I
3   H

18 Diagnosis of psychotic disorders

1   H
2   D
3   B

19 Laboratory investigations to assist psychiatric diagnosis and management

1   D
2   I
3   J

20 Assessing suicidal intent/risk

1   D, G, I
2   A, C
3   A, C, G

21 Physical examination of patients presenting with self-poisoning

1   D, G, K
2   B, D, K
3   A, I, L

22 Physical examination of patients presenting with self-poisoning

1   L, J
2   B, J, D
3   F, K, E

23 Physical examination of patients presenting with self-poisoning

1   D, I, J
2   L, H, G
3   L, H, G

24 Managing suicidal risk in the accident and emergency department

1   G
2   I
3   B

25 Managing suicidal risk in the accident and emergency department

1   A
2   C
3   F

26 Significant history in confirming a psychiatric diagnosis in deliberate self-harm

1   E
2   D
3   G

27 Significant history in confirming a psychiatric diagnosis in deliberate self-harm

1   B
2   A
3   I

28 Assessing suicidal risk

1   C
2   E
3   F

29 Investigations in patients suffering from acute and chronic confusional states

1   E
2   J
3   G

30 Investigations in patients suffering from acute and chronic confusional states

1   H
2   I
3   F

31 Differential diagnosis of psychotic disorders

1   F
2   A
3   D

32 Diagnosis of common mental disorders

1   I
2   D
3   J

33 Identification of signs and symptoms in a mental state examination

1   D
2   C
3   G

34 Identification of signs and symptoms in a mental state examination

1   A
2   D
3   H

35 Patient interviewing techniques

1   F
2   C
3   A

36 Application of patient interviewing techniques

1   B
2   F
3   A

37 Application of patient interviewing techniques

1   E
2   C
3   C

38 Application of patient interviewing techniques

1   B
2   D
3   G

39 Clinical applications of interviewing techniques

1   B
2   A
3   E

40 Differential diagnosis of psychosomatic syndromes

1   B
2   H
3   F

41 Differential diagnosis of anxiety disorders

1   G
2   C
3   H

42 Differential diagnosis of mood disorders

1   F
2   G
3   B

43 Mechanisms of adverse drug interactions

1   C, D
2   E, I
3   B

44 Identification of drug interactions

1   A, D, F
2   B, G, K
3   E, I, J

45 Differential diagnosis of somatoform disorders

1   C
2   D, E
3   A, G

46 Differential diagnosis of psychotic disorders

1   D
2   H
3   F

47 Risk factors for mental illness in older people

1   B, F, H
2   B, F
3   B, C, F

48 Differential diagnosis of mental disorders presenting with physical symptoms

1   C
2   C, H
3   D

49 Differential diagnosis of mood disorders

1   F, H
2   F
3   C

50 Differential diagnosis of anxiety disorders

1   D, E
2   D
3   B, E

FURTHER READING

General textbooks

Buckley P, Bird J, Harrison G, Prewette G (2004) *Examination Notes in Psychiatry*, 4th edn. London: Hodder Arnold.

Gelder M, Mayou R, Cowen P (2004) *Shorter Oxford Textbook of Psychiatry*, 4th edn. Oxford: Oxford University Press.

Gelder MG, Lopez-Ibor J Jr, Andreasen NC (2003) *New Oxford Textbook of Psychiatry*. Oxford: Oxford University Press.

Sadock BJ, Sadock VA (2005) *Kaplan and Sadock's Comprehensive Textbook of Psychiatry*, 7th edn. Philadelphia: Lippincott Williams & Wilkins.

Johnstone E, Lawrie S, Owens D, Sharpe MD (2004) *Companion to Psychiatric Studies*, 7th edn. London: Churchill Livingstone.

Puri BK, Hall AD (2004) *Revision Notes in Psychiatry*, 2nd edn. London: Hodder Arnold.

Paykel ES (1992) *Handbook of Affective Disorders*, 2nd edn. Edinburgh: Churchill Livingstone.

Thornicroft G, Szmukler G (2001) *Textbook of Community Psychiatry*. Oxford: Oxford University Press.

General adult psychiatry

Stein G, Wilkinson G (1998) *Seminars in General Adult Psychiatry*. Vols 1 and 2. London: Gaskell.

Old age psychiatry/organic psychiatry

Butler R, Pitt B (1998) *Seminars in Old Age Psychiatry*. London: Gaskell.

Lishman WA (1998) *Organic Psychiatry: The Psychological Consequences of Cerebral Disorder*, 3rd edn. Oxford: Blackwell Scientific.

Jacoby R, Oppenheimer C, eds (2002) *Psychiatry in the Elderly*, 3rd edn. Oxford: Oxford University Press.

Descriptive psychopathology

Hamilton M (1985) *Fish's Clinical Psychopathology: Signs and Symptoms in Psychiatry*, 2nd edn. Bristol: John Wright.

Sims A (2002) *Symptoms in Mind: An Introduction to Descriptive Psychopathology*, 3rd edn. London: Baillière Tindall.

Dynamic psychopathology/psychoanalysis

Edelson M (1990) *Psychoanalysis: A Theory in Crisis*. Chicago: University of Chicago Press.

Psychotherapy

Bateman A, Holmes J (2000) *Introduction to Psychotherapy: An Outline of Psychodynamic Principles and Practice*, 3rd edn. London: Routledge.
Greenberger D, Padesky C (1995) *Clinician's Guide to Mind Over Mood*. New York: Guilford Press.
Hawton K, Salkovskis PM, Kirk J, Clark DM, eds (2000) *Cognitive–behavioural Approaches for Adult Psychiatric Disorders: A Practical Guide*, 2nd edn. Oxford: Oxford University Press.

Psychology

Colman AM (2003) *Oxford Dictionary of Psychology*. Oxford: Oxford University Press.
Gupta D, Gupta R, eds (2003) *Psychology for Psychiatrists*. London: Whurr Publishers.
Munafo M (2002) *Psychology for the MRCPsych*, 2nd edn. London: Hodder Arnold.
Smith EE, Nolen-Hoeksema S, Fredrickson B, Loftus G (2003) *Atkinson and Hilgard's Introduction to Psychology*, 14th edn. USA: Wadsworth.
Tantam D, Birchwood M (1994) *Seminars in Psychology and Social Sciences*. London: Gaskell.

Basic sciences

Malhi G, Malhi S (2006) *Examination Notes in Psychiatry: Basic Sciences*, 2nd edn. London: Hodder Arnold.
Morgan G, Butler S (1993) *Seminars in Basic Neurosciences*. London: Gaskell.
Puri BK, Tyrer P (1998) *Sciences Basic to Psychiatry*, 2nd edn. London: Churchill Livingstone.
Weller M et al. (1991) *The Scientific Basis of Psychiatry*. London: WB Saunders.

Psychopharmacology

Anderson IM, Reid IC (2004) *Fundamentals of Clinical Psychopharmacology*, 2nd edn. London: Taylor and Francis.
Bazire S (2005) *Psychotropic Drug Directory: The Professionals Pocket. Handbook and Aide Mémoire*. Philadelphia: Lippincott, Williams & Wilkins.
Cookson J, Taylor D, Katona C (2002) *Use of Drugs in Psychiatry*, 5th edn. London: Gaskell.
King D, ed. (2004) *Seminars in Clinical Psychopharmacology*, 2nd edn. London: Gaskell.
Mehta DK, ed. (2005) *British National Formulary*. Oxon: Pharmaceutical Press.
Stahl S (2000) *Essential Psychopharmacology: Neuroscientific Basis and Practical Applications*, 2nd edn. Cambridge: Cambridge University Press.
Taylor D, Paton C, Kerwin R. (2005) *The Maudsley 2005–2006 Prescribing Guidelines*, 8th edn. London: Taylor and Francis.

Classification

American Psychiatric Association (1994) *Diagnostic and Statistical Manual of Mental Disorders: DSM-IV*, 4th edn. Washington, DC: APA.

World Health Organization (1992) *The ICD-10 Classification of Mental and Behavioural Disorders: Clinical Descriptions and Diagnostic Guidelines*. World Health Organization, Geneva.

OSCEs

Boom JVD, Tony J, Thirumalai S. (2004) *Objective Structured Clinical Examination for Psychiatric Trainees*, Vol II. Quay Books, MA: Healthcare Limited.

Boom, JVD, Tony J, Thirumalai S. (2003) *Objective Structured Clinical Examination for Psychiatric Trainees*, Vol I. Quay Books, MA: Healthcare Limited.

Michael Albert, ed. (2004) *OSCEs in Psychiatry*. London: Churchill Livingstone.

Ranga Rao, ed. (2005) *OSCEs in Psychiatry*. London: Gaskell.

INDEX

Note: Italicised page numbers are for section 1 (a guide to MRCPsych Part I examination). References for ISQs (papers 1–6) are given in the form of the starting page number followed in curled brackets by the question number(s) which may runover on to the following page(s). References for EMIs (paper 7) are distinguished from the ISQs by use of square brackets. A few indexed topics are mentioned just in the answer.

abstraction
  arbitrary   100(18)
  selective   100(20)
accident and emergency department, suicide
    risk management   194–5[24–5]
accommodation, visual, drugs adversely
    affecting   34(94–8)
acquisition stage of conditioning   99(10)
action potentials   56(78–80)
admission, compulsory, under Mental Health
    Act   194[24]
adrenaline   78(49)
adventitious reinforcement   54(37)
adverse drug reactions
  EMIs   213–14[43–4]
  ISQs   5
    individual questions   33(83–98),
      56(82–100), 78(62–82), 103(67–76),
      152(68–87)
aetiology
  in EMIs of mental disorders   174[4]
  in ISQs   5
    classification of mental disorders based
      on   40(215–19)
    individual questions   39(205–14),
      61(180–9), 84(182–96),
      109(192–205), 157(190–200)
affect/mood
  assessment   111(232–5)
  perplexed   59(134)
  in schizophrenia   105(118–19), 156(157)
affective (mood) disorders   158(199–200),
    160(230–1)
  differential diagnosis   212[42], 219[49]
  ICD-10   87(232)
  mixed   160(232)
  see also anxiety; bipolar affective disorder;
      depression; schizoaffective disorder
agitation   160(232–4)

agonist   103(63)
  inverse   103(64), 127(67)
agoraphobia   42(249), 60(157), 76(21–5),
    109(197), 158(196)
agrammatism (jargon aphasia)   31(49)
alcohol
  abuse   40(213), 61(183), 81(111), 111(231),
      129(115), 176[6], 193[23], 194[24]
  depression and   153(101)
  hallucinosis   153(93–6), 155(133),
      201[31]
  history-taking/interviewing   111(231),
      134(218–22)
  ICD-10 and   40(225)
  withdrawal syndrome   181[11], 186[16]
  see also delirium tremens; Korsakoff's
      disease; Wernicke's encephalopathy
  metabolism   77(44)
alexithymia   154(112–16)
alpha-methyldopa, adverse reactions   78(59)
Alzheimer's disease   185[15]
  depression and   105(100)
  diagnosis   40(218)
    differential   180[10]
  emotional lability and   107(165)
  late paraphrenia and   105(111)
  mental state examination   42(254), 87(228),
      135(232)
  physical/neurological examination   65(260),
      135(238), 161(260)
  spatial disorientation and   155(134)
  suicide and   158(197)
ambitendency   173[3]
amino acids, excitatory, receptors   33(78–82)
amitriptyline, pharmacology (incl. adverse
    effects)   33(84), 127(72)
  overdose   192[22]
amnesia see dysmnesic syndrome; memory
    impairment

amphetamines 191[21]
  adverse reactions 78(60)
  drug screen 198[28]
amygdala, lesions 65(253)
anal stage of psychosexual development
    60(169), 77(36)
analgesics, drug screen 190[20], 198[28]
analytic psychotherapy 85(202–10)
anhedonia 59(146–50), 80(110), 104(93),
    156(158), 197[27]
ankle jerks, absent 65(256–60), 161(260)
anorexia nervosa 58(108), 80(93), 82(134–6,
    138), 105(122–6), 197[27]
  depression vs 104(87–91)
antagonists, competitive 127(66)
anticholinergic (antimuscarinic) drugs
  adverse reactions 79(73–77), 128(91–5)
  chlorpromazine and 102(51)
anticholinergic (antimuscarinic) effects of
    antipsychotics 150(41), 187[17]
antidepressants see monoamine oxidase
    inhibitors; serotonin reuptake inhibitors,
    selective; tricyclic antidepressants
antimanic drugs, serum levels 190[20]
antimuscarinic drugs and effects see
    anticholinergic drugs; anticholinergic
    effects
antipsychotics (neuroleptics), adverse reactions
    57(91–5)
antisocial behaviour in boys 125(49)
antisocial personality disorder (dissocial
    personality disorder) 85(195), 86(223),
    108(168), 158(205), 171[1], 172[2],
    196[26]
anxiety 59(126), 84(172–8), 108(187–91)
  in post-traumatic stress syndrome 80(109)
  psychoanalytic theory 108(187–96)
  vitamin B$_{12}$ deficiency and 105(102)
  see also fears
anxiety disorders/states
  cognitive model 53(21–5)
  depression comorbid with 220[50]
  differential diagnosis 178[8], 211[41],
    220[50]
  generalized 42(252), 83(156), 104(82–6),
    159(212), 211[41], 220[50]
  psychodynamic factors 156(176–80)
  see also specific anxiety disorders
aphasia 160(242)
  Broca's 31(44)

  jargon 31(49)
  Wernicke's 31(48)
arbitrary abstraction 100(18)
arson (fire setting) 150(46)
assimilation 149(30)
associative learning 99(8–9)
attachment 32(56–8), 54(52–6), 125(48)
attention 135(231–35)
  divided, flexibility 76(13)
  selective 148(1–5)
  stage models 76(14)
attention deficit hyperactivity disorder
    110(206), 150(48)
attribution theory 29(12, 16), 123(13–15)
audible thoughts 204[34]
auditory hallucinations 36(129–30, 132–3),
    60(154), 80(105), 106(142), 129(126),
    159(214)
  paranoid psychosis with, drug misuse and
    39(210–14)
aura of complex partial seizures 161(255–9)
autism 62(193)
autochonous delusions 37(164), 154(121–2)
automatic obedience 173[3]
automatic thoughts, negative 100(18–22)
autoscopy 60(153), 80(103–8), 155(141–5)
aversive conditioning 54(36), 99(13)
avoidance learning/training/conditioning
    84(182–6), 85(190), 148(6)
avoidant personality disorder 172[2]

Babcock sentence 64(232)
backward conditioning 29(13)
bacterial septicaemia 176[6]
barbiturates 39(210)
Beck's Depression Inventory 154(113),
    190[20]
Beck's depressive triad 30(36)
bedwetting (nocturnal enuresis) 84(182)
behavioural psychology
  in curriculum 6
  in ISQs 5
    individual questions 30(34–41),
      53(21–37), 76(16–32), 100(23–32),
      124(21–35), 148(13–24)
behavioural therapy 124(21–5)
  spasmodic torticollis 136(257)
beliefs
  dysfunctional 148(11)
  false 37(167)

Bell's palsy 64(241–5)
Bender Gestalt test 29(15)
Benton Verbal Fluency Test 101(33)
Benton Visual Retention Test 149(26)
benzodiazepines 127(73), 152(78–7)
    antagonist 127(67)
    cognitive impairment 61(184)
    overdose 193[23], 195[25]
    pharmacology 32(68–77), 55(63–7), 103(60)
    receptors 103(62, 64), 151(58)
    tolerance 152(78–82)
    withdrawal syndrome 152(83–7)
benztropine, adverse effects 34(98)
bereavement 61(189), 106(134), 109(193)
    grief reaction 35(109–13), 36(139–43),
        80(94), 130(149), 153(102–6)
bias, self-serving 99(4)
Bibring, Edward 60(172)
bingeing see bulimia nervosa
bioavailability 32(69), 78(46–7)
bipolar affective disorder 188[18], 212[42]
    characteristic features 63(238), 107(163)
    denial and 108(167)
    drug abuse and 42(245)
    rapid cycling 135(228–30)
birth and anxiety 109(192)
Bleuler's criteria and schizophrenia 133(201),
        158(201)
blood–brain barrier
    dopamine and 56(71)
    psychotropic drugs and 102(50), 103(66)
blushing, fear of 129(111–15)
body image disturbances 82(147), 197[27]
Bonnet's syndrome 181[11]
borderline personality disorder 87(236–40),
        106(132), 110(209), 197[27], 219[49]
Bowlby, John 32(58), 54(52–4), 125(41)
brain imaging 136(241–5), 199[29]
brainstem lesions 88(251–5)
breast-feeding, drugs to avoid 33(84–8)
Briquet's syndrome 40(219), 215[45]
Broca's aphasia 31(44)
bulimia nervosa (bingeing; hyperphagia;
        overeating) 36(149–58), 58(106–10),
        80(97), 82(137), 82(147–56), 132(183–7)
    history-taking, example 24
buspirone 101(43), 127(75)

Cambridge Cognitive Battery (CAMCOG)
    160(240)

cannabis 40(212), 192[22]
Cannon–Bard theory 30(26)
Capgras' syndrome 130(141–5), 201[31]
carbamazepine 150(38)
    adverse effects 33(86), 34(90), 57(96)
castration anxiety 84(176), 109(194),
        157(178)
catalepsy 130(131)
cataplexy 59(137), 130(134), 183[13]
catatonia 34(99–103), 58(111–15), 173[3]
categorical classification, relative merits
        134(208)
categorization 100(22)
Category Test 54(41)
caudate nucleus lesions 136(251)
cause see aetiology
cerebellar disease 161(250)
cerebral hypoxia 174[4], 186[16]
Charles Bonnet syndrome 181[11]
children
    development see development
    school refusal 150(47)
    separation anxiety 84(177), 109(195)
    sexual abuse 157(191)
    sick role behaviour 76(16–20)
    see also infant
chlordiazepoxide, adversely effects 34(94)
chloride channels, GABA receptors 103(60),
        151(60–1)
chlorpromazine 77(38–42), 102(51–5)
    neuroleptic dose equivalents 57(97)
chronic fatigue syndrome 58(122),
        210[40]
cimetidine, adverse reactions 78(62)
circumstantiality 155(151–5)
citalopram 101(42), 149(31)
clang associations 128(98)
clarification 205[35], 206[36], 209[39]
classification and diagnosis in ISQs 5
    individual questions 40(215–29),
        62(190–204), 85(197–201), 87(231–40),
        110(206–20), 133(193–212),
        158(201–15)
clinical theory and skills
    in curriculum 8
    in ISQs 5
        individual questions 39(205–60),
            61(180–260), 84(182–260),
            132(178–92), 157(190–261)
    see also specific skills

closed question 206[36], 207[37], 208[38], 209[39]
clouding of consciousness 59(131–5), 104(78)
clozapine 150(51)
   diabetes mellitus and 126(62–3)
   hypersalivation 126(60)
cocaine 81(123)
   overdose 193[23]
cognition
   defining 124(17–18)
   neuroleptic effects 126(64–5), 150(42–3)
cognitive–behavioural model of depression
   29(11), 30(34–7), 53(26–30)
cognitive development 32(59–63), 55(57–61)
cognitive dissonance 30(31–3), 99(1–2)
cognitive estimates test 87(226)
cognitive impairment
   causes 61(180–4)
   testing for (mental state examination)
     63(238–40), 87(229), 160(240–9)
cognitive learning theory 124(19)
cognitive model of anxiety 53(21–5)
cognitive theory 29(6–10)
   assimilation in 149(30)
   panic disorder 124(26–30)
cognitive triad of depression 30(38)
communication skills *16*, *19–20*
   examples *23*
community mental health team, referral to
   194[24]
competitive antagonists 127(66)
compulsory admission under Mental Health
   Act 194[24]
computed tomography 136(241–5)
concentration tests 42(246, 251), 87(227)
concrete operational stage of cognitive
   development 32(63), 55(60–1)
conditioning 75(8–10)
   acquisition stage 99(10)
   aversive 54(36), 99(13)
   avoidance (avoidance learning/training)
     84(182–6), 85(190), 148(6)
   backward 29(13)
   classical 29(13), 30(18, 28), 75(10), 99(8)
   instrumental 75(1), 77(32)
   operant 99(9), 148(6–10)
   Pavlovian 75(2)
   primary reward 100(28)
   second order 100(27)
   two-step process 53(16–20)

confabulation 104(77–81), 129(119), 155(129), 156(160)
confidentiality 112(248)
confusional states (acute and chronic)
   differential diagnosis/causes 180[10], 184[14], 186[16], 187[17]
   identification of signs and symptoms 176[6]
   investigations 177[7], 199–200[29–30]
consciousness, clouding 59(131–5), 104(78)
consent
   capacity to, assessment, example *25*
   to ECT *23*
control, delusion of 156(159)
conversion disorders 158(195), 215[45], 218[48]
   hysterical 35(114–18), 83(162–6)
cortical lesion 88(251–5)
corticosteroids, adverse reactions 78(61)
cortisol and mood disorders 158(200)
countertransference 37(177–8), 131(160), 156(165)
covert sensitization 84(188)
creatinine kinase 189[19]
Creutzveldt–Jakob disease 80(98)
curriculum outline *6–8*

darkness, fear of 125(44)
date, misidentification 63(231)
de Clérambault syndrome 83(158)
defence mechanisms 60(155–7, 159–64), 61(179), 130(146–50), 149(50)
   ego 38(180–4), 60(157), 83(162–6), 84(172–5), 129(106, 108), 156(162–5, 174), 175[5]
   in hysterical conversion disorder 83(162–6)
   in neuroses 60(160, 162–3)
   in obsessive–compulsive disorder 38(180–4), 130(147)
   in phobias 60(155–7, 159)
déjà vu 155(148)
delirium 158(198), 202[32]
delirium tremens 40(215), 42(250), 81(127), 107(162)
delusion(s) 35(124–8), 36(130–1), 83(161), 106(144), 129(125)
   autochonous 37(164), 154(121–2)
   of control 156(159)
   of double 144
   explaining to patient 112(250)

persecutory/paranoid 196[26]
  alcohol abuse 153(94)
delusional disorder 218[48]
  persistent 201[31]
dementia
  differential diagnosis/causes 182[12],
      185[15]
  frontal lobe type 101(38)
  multi-infarct/vascular 161(244), 184[14],
      187[17]
  prion 80(98–102)
  pseudodementia vs 160(241)
  see also Alzheimer's disease
denial 80(93–7), 83(166), 108(167–71),
    130(146), 175[5]
  in grief reaction 35(111), 36(139), 80(94)
dependent personality disorder 171[1]
depersonalization and derealization
    58(116–18, 123), 59(126–30), 82(146),
    155(142, 146)
depolarization 56(77–8, 80)
depression 104(87–101)
  anxiety comorbid with 220[50]
  cognitive–behavioural model 29(11),
      30(34–7), 53(26–30)
  cognitive impairment 61(182)
  cognitive triad 30(38)
  defence mechanisms 130(150)
  denial in 80(95)
  diagnosis 153(97–101), 184[14], 197[27],
      212[42], 219[49], 220[50]
    elderly 181[11]
    ICD-10 and 40(226)
  drug-induced 78(58–62)
  eating disorders and 104(87–91), 132(187)
  life events and 155(136–40)
  mental state examination 42(255),
      63(233–7), 135(233), 203[33]
  post-psychotic 62(190)
  postnatal, history-taking, example 24
  psychodynamic theories 60(170–4)
  psychosexual history in severe depression
      63(209), 160(236)
  schizoaffective disorder and 85(199)
  sexual function in 104(96), 109(204)
  symptoms/features 37(153), 58(120–1),
      59(129), 82(133), 83(155), 104(92–6),
      197[27]
  severe/major depression 59(144), 212[42],
      219[49]

somatic 220[50]
  vitamin B$_{12}$ deficiency and 105(106)
  see also bipolar affective disorder
derealization and depersonalization
    58(116–18, 122), 59(126–30), 82(146),
    155(142, 146)
descriptive psychopathology
  in curriculum 7
  in ISQs 5
    individual questions 34(99–169),
        57(101–54), 79(83–161), 104(77–166),
        128(96–145), 153(88–160)
development, human/child
  in curriculum 5–6
  in ISQs 5
    individual questions 31(52–63),
        54(50–61), 77(35–7), 101(39–41),
        125(39–50), 149(28–30)
diabetes mellitus 82(154)
  antipsychotics and 126(62–3), 150(52)
diagnosis see classification and diagnosis
Diagnostic and Statistical Manual-IV
    87(236–40), 133(203–7)
  ICD-10 compared with 62(190–4)
  schizophrenia 133(198), 158(206–10)
diazepam
  adverse effects 34(92)
    overdose 193[23], 195[25]
  pharmacokinetics 32(68), 33(71–2)
dichotomous reasoning 100(21)
direct question 205[35]
disorientation, spatial 155(131–5)
dissocial (antisocial) personality disorder
    86(223), 108(168), 158(205), 171[1],
    172[2], 196[26]
dissociation/dissociative states 82(142–6),
    109(201), 110(211–15), 130(131–5, 141,
    147), 135(231), 215[45]
distribution volume 55(64, 68–70)
dopamine 56(70), 126(58–9)
  receptors 78(51–5), 127(69)
    agonists 127(71)
    antagonists 102(56), 213[43]
doppelganger phenomenon (autoscopy)
    60(153), 80(103–8), 155(141–5)
dothiepin (dosulepin), adverse effects 34(95),
    103(68), 213[43]
dream(s) 61(178), 83(167–8)
dream work/analysis 84(170, 181), 85(206),
    108(178), 157(186)

droperidol 77(39)

drug abuse 39(210–14)
    bipolar affective disorder and 42(245)
    ICD-10 and 40(225)
    poisoning 191[21]
    see also specific drugs

drug overdose 190[20], 192–3[22–3], 195[25]

drug therapy *see* psychopharmacology

DSM-IV *see* Diagnostic and Statistical
    Manual-IV

dynamic psychopathology
    in curriculum 7
    in ISQs 5
        individual questions 37(170–204),
            60(155–79), 83(162–81), 108(167–91),
            130(146–77), 156(161–89)

dysarthria 136(247)

dysmnesic syndrome 133(188–92)
    see also Korsakoff's disease

dysphasia 88(257)
    receptive 160(238)
    subcortico-motor 160(237)

dysphoria 156(158)

dystonia 183[13]

eating disorders 36(149–58), 58(106–10),
    80(93, 97), 82(133–41), 82(147–56),
    104(87–91), 105(122–6), 132(183–7),
    197[27]

echolalia 59(136)

echopraxia 59(140), 135(237)

ECT, consent 23

effect, Thorndike's law of 99(11)

ego 35(125), 38(186), 60(165), 83(169),
    84(170), 101(39), 108(172, 174, 176),
    131(166–70), 132(171, 174–6),
    156(166–75)
    anxiety and 109(190)
    defence mechanisms 38(180–4), 60(157),
        83(162–6), 84(172–5), 129(106, 108),
        156(162–5), 156(174), 175[5]
    functions 156(171–5)
    strength 156(166–70)

eidetic images 36(134–8)

ejaculation, premature 84(185)

elderly/older people
    cognitive testing 160(240–4)
    psychiatric diagnosis 181[11]
    risk factors for mental illness 217[47]
    self-harm 61(185–9)

Electra complex 60(167)

electroconvulsive therapy (ECT),
    consent 23

Ellis, Albert 30(34)

emergency management *16, 22*

EMIs *see* extended matching items

emotional lability/instability 107(162–6),
    112(254)
    personality disorder with 171[1]

empathy, expressing 207[37], 208[38]

encoding, visual imagery during 30(21),
    123(7)

enuresis, nocturnal 84(182)

epilepsy, temporal lobe 81(127)
    see also seizures

epinephrine (adrenaline) 78(49)

epinosic gain 130(151–5)

equipment use *16, 21–2*

Erikson, Erik 77(37), 101(39)

examination in ISQs *see* mental state
    examination; physical examination

excitatory neurotransmitters 56(81)
    receptors 33(78–82)

exhibitionism 84(186)

experiences, human, normal 129(121–5),
    155(146–50)

extended matching items (EMIs) *3*
    in context of clinical management *10–11*
    format *9–10*
    frequently used terms *12*
    marking *11*
    reasons for introduction of *10*
    skills and knowledge tested in *10*
    tackling *11*
    time and marking system *3*

extinction 75(8–9)

falling from height, fear 125(44)

false beliefs 37(167)

family and relatives
    dynamics, interviewing about 86(219)
    schizophrenia explained to *23*
    see also maternal deprivation; parent–
        infant behaviour

fasciculations 161(252)

fears
    of blushing 129(111–15)
    children's 125(44–5), 126(50)
    of harmless objects, irrational 155(149)
    see also anxiety

feelings, patient's, objective evidence in
  interview 41(230–4)
fetishism 109(200)
fire setting 150(46)
first-rank symptoms 105(112–16), 106(142–6),
  128(99), 133(199), 153(98), 158(206)
flight of ideas 81(113–17), 156(156), 203[33]
flumazenil 127(67)
fluoxetine 150(35)
  adverse effects 34(89), 103(70), 214[44]
fluspirilene 150(39)
fluvoxamine, adverse effects 57(98), 103(71)
Freud, Sigmund 38(185–9), 39(195–9),
  60(165–9), 83(167–71), 84(181)
  psychoanalytic theory 83(167–71), 84(181),
    108(172–6)
frontal lobe dementia 182[2], 185[15]
frontal lobe function
  assessment 87(225), 149(27)
    example 25
  impaired 88(247–50), 101(35, 37–8)
fugue states 80(96), 215[45]
functional behavioural analysis 124(23),
  124(31–5), 148(13–16)

GABA (gamma-aminobutyric acid) 78(48),
  127(73)
  receptors 78(56–7), 103(61), 127(70, 73),
    151(58–62)
    chloride channels 103(60), 151(60–1)
gamma-aminobutyric acid see GABA
Ganser's syndrome 82(145), 110(212),
  155(135, 152)
gedankenlautwerden 34(102), 105(116)
General Health Questionnaire 86(215)
general practitioner, referral for follow-up to
  194[24]
generalized anxiety (disorder) 42(252),
  83(156), 104(82–6), 159(212), 211[41],
  220[50]
Gerstmann–Sträussler syndrome 80(99)
Gerstmann syndrome 88(256–60)
Gilles de la Tourette syndrome 150(44)
globoid cell leukodystrophy (Krabbe's disease)
  80(102)
globus pallidus lesions 136(255)
glutamate 78(50)
  receptors 33(81)
glycine 78(48)
  receptors 33(81)

grief reaction 35(109–13), 36(139–43), 80(94),
  130(149), 153(102–6)
Guillain–Barré syndrome 65(258)
gustatory hallucinations 129(127)

habituation 30(29–30), 76(26)
Hachinski Scale 161(244)
hallucinations 36(129–34), 59(151–4),
  129(126–30)
  alcohol abuse 153(93–6), 155(193), 201[31]
  auditory see auditory hallucinations
  gustatory 129(127)
  Lilliputian 37(169)
  reflex 179[9]
  tactile/haptic 36(131), 79(84), 81(123–7),
    179[9]
  visual 35(110), 59(133), 60(153), 80(103),
    106(130), 129(128)
  see also pseudohallucinations
halo effect 100(16)
haloperidol 77(42)
  adverse reactions 33(83), 79(78), 103(73)
  pharmacokinetics 56(70)
Halstead Category test 31(42)
Halstead–Reitan Neurological Battery 31(45),
  101(34)
haptic (tactile) hallucinations 36(131), 79(84),
  81(123–7), 179[9]
Hawthorne effect 100(17)
height, fear of falling from 125(44)
helplessness, learned 30(28), 53(28, 31–5),
  75(3–7), 85(189), 100(24), 124(16–17)
hepatic failure
  confusion 176[6]
  drugs contraindicated in 57(96–100),
    79(78–82)
hepatic function tests 190[20]
history-taking and interviewing 16, 20–1
  in EMIs 205–9[35–9]
  examples 24
  in ISQs 5
    individual questions 41(230–42),
      62(205–22), 85(202–23), 110(221–40),
      134(213–30), 159(216–39)
    on technique 41(235–9), 63(210–14)
histrionic personality disorder 81(128–32),
  107(164), 158(204)
human development see development
Huntington's chorea/disease 65(256), 182[12],
  216[46]

hydrocephalus, normal pressure 185[15]
8-hydroxydipropylamine-tetralin (8–OH–
    DPAT) 151(63)
5-hydroxytryptamine and its receptors etc. *see*
    serotonin
hyperphagia *see* bulimia nervosa
hyperpolarization 56(79)
hyperprolactinaemia 126(61)
hypersalivation 126(58–60)
hypnagogic states 106(132), 106(136), 129(129)
hypnopompic states 106(136), 129(130)
hypnosis 85(204)
hypochondriasis 59(141–5), 110(215), 210[40],
    215[45]
hypomania 63(215), 196[26]
hypothalamic lesions 81(115), 136(254)
    see also limbic hypothalamic–pituitary–
        adrenal complex
hypoxia, cerebral 174[4], 186[16]
hysteria 80(106)
    ICD-10 and 62(198)
hysterical amnesia 130(135)
hysterical conversion syndrome/disorder
    35(114–18), 83(162–6)
hysterical (histrionic) personality 81(128–32),
    107(164), 158(204)

ICD-10 40(225–9)
id 38(185, 187, 189), 39(195–7, 199), 60(166,
    168), 108(173), 131(167), 132(175), 157(189)
id anxiety 84(178)
ideas
    flight of 81(113–17), 156(156), 203[33]
    of reference 129(123)
identification 83(162)
    projective 156(161–5)
    see also misidentification
imprinting 30(27), 100(23)
inattention, selective, lack 135(231–5)
incubation 76(27), 100(26)
individual statement questions (ISQs) *3, 9*
    frequently used terms *12*
    outline (topics covered) *5*
    preparing for and tackling *9*
    time and marking system *3*
infant
    paranoid–schizoid position 37(165–6)
    parent and, normal interactive behaviour
        101(40)
    see also children

information
    processing 148(1–5)
    retrieval from memory 30(21), 123(6–8)
innominate substance lesions 136(252)
insight 204[34]
instinct and instinctual behaviour 108(175),
    123(11)
instrumental conditioning 75(1), 77(32)
intellectual (cognitive) development
    32(59–63), 55(57–61)
International Classification of Diseases (ICD-
    10) 40(225–9), 62(190–204), 81(128–32),
    87(231–5), 133(193–7)
    DSM-IV compared with 62(190–4)
    personality disorders 171[1]
    schizophrenia 133(200), 158(206–15)
interpretation 206[36], 207[37], 209[39]
interviewer's behaviour 41(240–3), 86(220–1)
interviewing *see* history-taking and
    interviewing
ischaemic attacks, transient 187[17]
ISQs *see* individual statement questions

jargon aphasia 31(49)
Jung, Carl 108(177–86)

Klein, Melanie 52(12, 15), 60(170), 131(168)
Kleine–Levin syndrome 58(107)
Klüver–Bucy syndrome 58(106)
knee jerks, absent 65(256–60), 161(260)
Korsakoff's disease/psychosis/syndrome 40(7),
    81(124), 104(77), 155(132)
    see also dysmnesic syndrome
Krabbe's disease 80(102)
kuru 80(101)

laboratory tests 189[19]
    confusional states 177[7], 199[29], 200[30]
learned helplessness 30(28), 53(28, 31–5),
    75(3–7), 85(189), 100(24), 124(16–17)
learning
    associative 99(8–9)
    cognitive 124(19)
    observational 149(17–21)
    secondary reward 100(29)
    theories of 29(17), 31(39), 99(12–15),
        100(30–2), 109(197–201), 149(22, 24)
    see also conditioning
learning disability *see* mental retardation
Lewy body disease 80(100), 182[12]

life events and depression 155(136–40)
Lilliputian hallucinations 37(169)
limbic hypothalamic–pituitary–adrenal
    complex 158(199)
lithium (lithium carbonate etc.)
  adverse effects 33(87), 79(72, 82),
      127(76–80), 214[44]
    overdose 192[22]
  past history of use 85(200)
  pharmacodynamics 102(59), 127(74)
liver see entries under hepatic
lofepramine, adverse effects 57(100)
lorazepam 127(73)
loxapine 150(36)
LSD 40(214), 58(124)
Luria–Nebraska battery test 31(46)
lysergic acid diethylamide 40(214), 58(124)

'magic' mushrooms 191[21]
magnetic resonance imaging 199[29]
Mahler, Margaret 125(42–3)
malingering 35(119–23), 82(142)
mammillary body lesions 65(254)
mania 58(125), 81(113), 154(107–11)
  schizophrenia and
      differential diagnosis 154(117–20)
      past history of 85(201)
  see also antimanic drugs; bipolar affective
      disorder; hypomania
maprotiline 101(45)
masturbation, childhood 101(41)
maternal deprivation/absence 109(196),
    149(28)
Meige's syndrome 161(254)
memory 99(7)
  long-term 30(23), 42(248)
  modal model 30(23)
  panoramic 129(124)
  procedural 30(24)
  retrieval of information 30(21), 123(6–8)
  short-term 30(23), 42(246), 63(228–9),
      76(15), 123(1–4, 11)
memory impairment/loss (amnesia)
  anterograde 104(80)
  dissociative 215[45]
  organic brain disease 65(251–5), 101(35–6),
      136(246, 251–5)
  psychogenic 31(51)
  short-term memory loss 88(246)
    vitamin B_{12} deficiency and 105(106)

  see also dysmnesic syndrome; hysterical
      amnesia
Mental Health Act
  assessment in context of 24
  compulsory admission 194[24]
mental retardation (learning disability)
    156(155)
  mild, in DSM-IV 110(207)
mental state examination
  EMIs 203–4[33–4]
  ISQs 5
    history-taking after 135(223)
    individual questions 42(246–55),
        63(223–40), 86(217), 87(224–30),
        111(241–50), 135(231–5), 160(240–9)
  see also Mini-Mental State Examination
N-methyl-D-aspartate receptors 33(78–80),
    151(59)
methyldopa, adverse reactions 78(59)
micropsia 37(169)
Mini-Mental State Examination 200[30]
  dementia vs pseudodementia 160(242)
Minnesota Multiphasic Personality Inventory
    123(5), 161(243)
misidentification 83(156–61)
mitgehen 173[3]
mitmachen 34(101)
moclobemide 102(46, 58), 149(32)
  adverse effects 34(91), 79(79), 103(72)
monoamine oxidase (MAO) inhibitors 102(46,
    57–8), 152(74–7)
months of year, reciting 42(246–55), 63(230)
mood, see also affect; affective disorder
motivation and motivational analysis
    124(20), 149(16)
motor (Broca's) aphasia 31(44)
motor (movement) disorders 135(236–40),
    183[13]
motor neurone(s), lower, disease/lesions of
    161(252)
motor neurone disease 65(258), 136(246–50)
movement (motor) disorders 135(236–40),
    183[13]
Mowerer's two-step conditioning process
    53(16–20)
multi-infarct (vascular) dementia 161(244),
    184[14], 187[17]
multiple personality disorder 110(214)
multiple sclerosis 127(68)
mushrooms, 'magic' 191[21]

narcissistic personality 62(194), 172[2]
narcolepsy 106(127–31)
near-death experiences 129(121)
negative automatic thoughts 100(18–22)
negative reinforcement 31(40), 99(12),
 101(32), 149(22, 24)
negative symptoms, schizophrenia
 105(117–21), 154(126–30)
nerve cell impulse conduction 56(77–81)
neurasthenia 110(213)
neuroimaging 136(241–5), 199[29]
neuroleptics (antipsychotics) 150(35–43)
 adverse/unwanted reactions 57(91–5),
  126(64–5), 127(71)
  anticholinergic/antimuscarinic effects
   150(41), 187[17]
 chlorpromazine dose equivalents 77(38–42)
 new generation 102(56)
 pharmacodynamics 150(35–43)
 pharmacokinetics 102(47–9, 51–5),
  126(64–5), 150(51–2)
neurological examination *see* physical (and
 neurological) examination
neuronal impulse conduction 56(77–81)
neuropsychology
 in curriculum 6
 in ISQs 5
  individual questions 31(42–51),
   54(38–49), 77(33–4), 101(33–8),
   125(36–8), 149(25–7)
neurosarcoidosis 216[46]
neuroses
 defence mechanisms 60(160, 162–3),
  84(174)
 dynamic psychotherapy in 38(192)
  brief 39(202)
 ICD-10 and 40(227), 87(233, 235), 133(197)
neurotoxic reactions 128(86–90)
neurotransmitters 56(72–6), 78(48–50)
 excitatory *see* excitatory neurotransmitters
 serotonergic synapses and 151(53–7)
night terrors 37(159–63), 106(131), 130(133)
NMDA receptors 33(78–80), 151(59)
nocturnal enuresis 84(182)
nomothetic approaches 30(18)
nortriptyline, sedative effect 103(75)

object relationships 52(11–15), 156(175)
Objective Structured Clinical Examination
 (OSCE) 3–4, 13–25

advantages and disadvantages 14
format 17
historical perspective 13–14
marking 3, 18
preparing for 19–22
problems with 14–15
skills tested 16
tackling 23–5
time 3
observational learning 149(17–21)
obsessional personality 34(104)
obsessive–compulsive disorder (incl.
 obsessional thoughts) 107(152–6),
 109(199), 153(88–92)
 aetiology/development 58(118), 77(36),
  84(184)
 defence mechanisms 38(180–4), 130(147)
 depression and 153(97)
 differential diagnosis 178[8]
occipital lobe functional assessment 149(26)
Oedipus complex/oedipal stage 60(158, 167),
 157(184)
olanzapine, pharmacology 126(61)
older people *see* elderly
ondansetron 151(66)
open-ended questions 86(216), 110(221–5),
 205[35]
operant conditioning 99(9), 148(6–10)
operational stage of cognitive development
 32(62)
 concrete 32(63), 55(60–1)
optic disc oedema 39(205–9)
oral stage of psychosexual development
 60(169)
orientation
 spatial, disturbances 155(131–5)
 tests 63(223–7)
OSCE *see* Objective Structured Clinical
 Examination
overdose 190[20], 192–3[22–3], 195[25]
overeating *see* bulimia nervosa
overgeneralization 100(19)

pain, psychological vs physical origin
 107(157–61)
panic disorder (panic anxiety and panic
 attacks) 59(130), 84(176, 178), 158(196)
 cognitive theory explanation 124(26–30)
 differential diagnosis 178[8], 211[41]
panoramic memory 129(124)

papilloedema 39(205–9)

paracetamol overdose 194[24], 195[25]

paranoia 130(148)

paranoid delusions *see* delusions

paranoid psychosis with auditory
  hallucinations, drug misuse and
  39(210–14)

paranoid–schizoid position 154(123)
  infant 37(165–6)

paranoid schizophrenia 83(160), 130(145)

paranosic gain 37(170–4)

paraphrenia, late 105(107–11), 110(210),
  188[18]

pareidolia 128(96)

parent–infant behaviour, normal 101(40)
  see also maternal deprivation

parietal lobe function
  assessment 125(38)
  impairment (and lesions causing) 65(255),
    149(25)

parkinsonism and Parkinson's disease
    61(181), 88(242), 135(239), 136(258),
    161(251)

Parkinson's disease 61(181), 88(242),
    135(239), 136(258)

paroxetine 150(34)
  adverse effects 57(99)
  discontinuation reaction 213[43]

passive–aggressive personality disorder
    62(194)

Pavlovian conditioning 75(2)

pericyazine 150(37)

persecutory delusions *see* delusions

perseveration 81(118–22), 129(116), 156(160)

personality
  premorbid 86(211–15, 218, 223)
  tests/assessment 86(211), 123(5, 9–10),
    161(243)

personality (disorders) 171–2[1, 2]
  avoidant 172[2]
  borderline 87(236–40), 106(132), 110(209),
    197[27], 219[49]
  dependent 171[1]
  dissocial/antisocial 85(195), 86(223),
    108(168), 171[1], 172[2], 196[26]
  emotionally unstable 171[1]
  histrionic 81(128–32), 107(164), 158(204)
  ICD-10 diagnosis 171[1]
  multiple 110(214)
  narcissistic 62(194), 172[2]
  obsessional *see* obsessive–compulsive
    disorder
  passive–aggressive 62(194)
  schizoid 131(136–40)

personality trait 30(20)

pharmacodynamics
  in curriculum *7*
  in ISQs *5*
    individual questions 33(78–82),
      56(72–81), 78(48–57), 102(56–66),
      151(53–67)

pharmacokinetics
  in curriculum *7*
  in ISQs *5*
    individual questions 32(68–77),
      55(62–71), 77(43–7), 102(47–55),
      150(50–2)

pharmacology *see* psychopharmacology

phencyclidine 191[21], 216[46]

phenelzine
  adverse reactions 79(68–72, 81), 103(67)
  pharmacodynamics 102(57)

phenomenology of mental disorders 179[9]

phenylbutazone 56(69)

phobias 54(44), 58(117), 202[32]
  aetiology 84(187–91)
  behavioural assessment 76(26–30)
  defence mechanisms 60(155–7, 159)
  specific, pathogenesis 100(23–7)
  see also specific phobias

physical (and neurological) examination in
    ISQs *5, 16, 21*
  example *25*
  individual questions 42(256–60),
    64(241–60), 88(241–60), 112(251–60),
    135(236–60), 161(250–60)

physical symptoms *see* somatic
    manifestations; somatoform disorders

Piaget, Jean 31(52–3), 32(59–63), 54(50–1),
    55(57–61), 77(35)

pica 150(45)

pimozide 77(40), 213[43]

placebo effect 126(51–5)

porphyria, acute intermittent 174[4]

positive reinforcement 76(31)

positron emission tomography 54(49)

postnatal period
  depression, history-taking, example *24*
  psychosis 155(131)

post-traumatic stress syndrome 80(109–12)

potassium channel blockers 127(68)
practical skills *16*, *21–2*
Prader–Willi syndrome 83(153)
premature ejaculation 84(185)
premorbid personality 86(211–15, 218, 223)
pre-operational stage of cognitive
        development 32(60), 55(57), 55(59)
preparedness 76(28), 84(187), 100(25)
pressure of speech 129(117), 156(156)
presynaptic inhibition 127(70)
primacy effect 30(22), 123(8)
prion dementia 80(98–102)
procedural memory 30(24)
prochlorperazine 150(40)
procyclidine 40(211)
projection 60(163), 175[5]
projective identification 156(161–5)
prolactin levels
    assessment 189[19]
    excess 126(61)
prosopagnosia 31(50)
pseudobulbar palsy 65(246–50)
pseudodementia vs dementia 160(241)
pseudohallucinations 80(88–92), 106(132–5)
psychic determinism 157(187–8)
psychoanalytic technique 85(202–10)
psychoanalytic theory
    of anxiety 108(187–96)
    classical/traditional 77(36), 83(167–71),
        84(181), 108(172–6)
psychogenic amnesia 31(51)
psychogenic pain vs physical pain
        107(157–61)
psychogenic spasmodic torticollis 136(260)
psychology, basic
    in curriculum *6*
    in ISQs *5*
        individual questions 29(1–33), 52(1–20),
            75(1–15), 100(1–22), 123(1–20),
            148(1–12)
    see also behavioural psychology;
            neuropsychology; social psychology
psychometric approach 54(45)
psychopathology
    in curriculum *7–8*
    in ISQs *5*
        individual questions 34(99–204),
            57(101–79), 104(77–191),
            128(96–177), 153(88–189)
psychopharmacology in ISQs *5*

    individual questions 32(64–98),
        55(62–100), 77(35–82), 79(83–181),
        101(42–76), 126(51–95), 149(31–87)
psychoses
    acute episodes 84(179), 132(177)
    classification/diagnosis 158(203), 188[18]
        differential diagnosis 201[31], 216[46]
        DSM-IV and 62(191)
        ICD-10 and 40(227), 62(191), 87(233,
            235), 133(197)
    cocaine 81(123)
    depression following 62(190)
    history-taking/interviewing 111(240),
        134(213–17)
    Korsakoff's 40(7), 81(124), 104(77)
    paranoid, with auditory hallucinations, drug
        misuse and 39(210–14)
    puerperal 155(131)
    serial sevens test 87(230)
    transient psychotic symptoms 197[27]
psychosexual development 60(169), 157(184)
    obsessive–compulsive disorder and 77(36)
psychosexual disorders 109(202–5)
psychosexual history 62(205–9)
    severe depression 63(309), 160(236)
psychotherapy, dynamic 38(191–4)
    brief 39(200–4)
psychotropic drugs, pharmacodynamics
        127(71–5)
puerperium *see* postnatal period
punch–drunk syndrome 65(256)
punishment 31(41), 99(13), 149(23)
    harmful retaliatory, anxious expectation
        84(176–7)

QT_c prolongation 150(49–50), 214[44]
questions
    closed 206[36], 207[37], 208[38], 209[39]
    direct 205[35]
    open-ended 86(216), 110(221–5), 205[35]

reasoning, dichotomous 100(21)
recapitulation 208[38]
receptive dysphasia 160(238)
receptor ligands 103(63–5), 127(66–7)
reflex(es), tendon, absent 65(256–60),
        161(260)
reflex hallucinations 179[9]
regression 61(176)
reinforcement 29(1–5), 99(14–15), 100(30–2)

adventitious 54(37)
  negative 31(40), 99(12), 101(32), 149(22,
    24)
  partial 99(3)
  positive 76(31)
  schedules of 52(6–10), 75(11), 124(25)
  vicarious 75(12)
relatives *see* family and relatives; parent–
    infant behaviour
Rennick's Repeatable Battery 54(47)
repression 61(179), 85(203), 108(188)
Research Diagnostic Criteria, schizophrenia
    133(202)
reward 75(11), 100(28–9)
Rey–Osterreith Figure Test 54(39)
risperidone
  adverse reactions 33(83), 34(93), 103(74),
    213[43]
  pharmacology 32(64–7), 126(57)
ritanserin 151(65)
Rorschach's test 99(5)
ruminations 128(101–5)

salivation, excessive 126(58–60)
sarcoidosis, neurological manifestations
    216[46]
schema 30(35)
schizoaffective disorder 81(115), 85(197–201)
schizoid, defining 131(161–5)
see also paranoid–schizoid position
schizoid personality 130(136–40)
schizophrenia 59(141)
  aetiology 132(178–82)
  characteristic/frequently-occurring features
    81(115), 104(81), 107(166), 128(96–100),
    155(154)
  classification/diagnosis 62(192),
    133(198–202), 158(201, 206–15),
    188[18], 202[32]
  delusional perception and 35(127)
  differential diagnosis 218[48], 219[49]
  explaining to relative 23
  history-taking/interviewing 41(244),
    160(239), 196[26]
  laboratory investigations 189[19]
  mania vs acute episode of 154(120)
  mental state examination 63(238–40),
    135(234)
  negative symptoms 105(117–21),
    154(126–30)

paranoid 83(160), 130(145)
  past/previous history of 105(109)
    and mania 85(201)
  physical/neurological examination
    136(240)
  physical symptoms 218[48]
  prodromal symptoms 128(104),
    158(210–15)
  suicide risk 36(144–8)
schizotypal disorders
  in DSM-IV 62(192), 110(208)
  in ICD-10 62(192)
Schneider, Carl 106(137–41)
Schneider, Kurt 106(141)
  first-rank symptoms 105(112–16),
    106(142–6), 128(99), 133(199), 153(98),
    158(206)
school refusal 150(47)
science, basic
  in curriculum 6–7
  in ISQs 5
    individual questions 29(1–53), 52(1–61),
      75(1–37), 99(1–41), 123(1–50),
      148(1–30)
sedative effect, unwanted 103(67–76)
seizures, complex partial 184[14]
  aura of 161(255–9)
  see also epilepsy
selective attention 148(1–5)
selective inattention, lack 135(231–5)
selective serotonin reuptake inhibitors *see*
    serotonin reuptake inhibitors
self-harm, deliberate 196–7[26–7]
  elderly 61(185–9)
  see also drug overdose; suicide
self-psychology 52(1–5)
self-serving bias 99(4)
sensorimotor stage of cognitive development
    32(59, 61), 55(58)
sensory aphasias (Wernicke's aphasia) 31(48)
sensory distortions 79(83–7)
separation anxiety 84(177), 109(195)
septicaemia, bacterial 176[6]
serial sevens test 87(226–30)
serotonergic synapses 151(53–7)
serotonin (5–HT) receptors 127(75),
    151(63–7)
  agonists 151(63)
  antagonists 102(56), 151(65–6)
  downregulation 213[43]

serotonin reuptake inhibitors, selective
57(87–90), 101(42–5), 149(31, 33–5)
   chlorpromazine and 102(52)
sertraline 149(33)
   adverse effects 34(88, 96), 103(75)
sexual abuse, childhood 157(191)
sexual behaviour 84(171)
   children 101(41)
   history-taking see psychosexual history
sexual dysfunction 109(202–5)
sick role behaviour 76(16–20)
side-effects see adverse drug reactions
sitting in interview, inability 63(215–19)
skills see clinical theory and skills
sleep disorders 37(159–63), 106(127–31),
   130(133–4)
social anxiety/phobia 59(143), 60(157, 159),
   82(140), 84(84), 109(198), 129(112)
   differential diagnosis 178[8], 211[41]
social psychology
   in curriculum 6
   in ISQs 5
somatic manifestations/physical
   manifestations of psychiatric disorders
   57(101–5)
   depression 220[50]
   differential diagnosis 218[48]
somatization and somatization disorder
   60(162), 157(190–4), 210[40]
somatoform disorders 59(145), 110(211), 215[45]
somnambulism 130(131)
spasmodic torticollis 136(256–60)
spatial disorientation 155(131–5)
speech, fluent 160(237)
speech disorders 88(241–6), 129(116–20),
   156(156)
   see also aphasia; dysarthria; dysphasia
Speech Sound Perception Test 125(38)
startle response 81(112)
stations in OSCEs 17
stereotypies 59(139), 81(120)
steroids, adverse reactions 78(61)
stranger anxiety 125(39–40), 149(28–9)
Stroop's (Color-Word Inference) Test 54(40),
   54(48), 77(34)
subcortico-motor dysphasia 160(237)
subdural haematoma, chronic 180[10]
sublimation 61(177), 83(163), 129(106–10)
substance abuse see drug abuse and specific
   drugs

substantia innominata lesions 136(252)
suicide
   attempted 85(192–6), 155(136)
   risk of 107(147–51)
   A & E department 194–5[24–5]
   Alzheimer's disease and 158(197)
   assessment 190[20], 198[28]
   schizophrenia and 36(144–8)
sulpiride 33(85), 77(41)
superego 38(188), 39(198), 83(168), 108(176),
   132(172–3, 175)
   anxiety and 108(189)
symptoms in classification of mental disorders
   40(220–3)
   see also somatic manifestations;
      somatization; somatoform disorders
synaesthesia 99(6)
syringobulbia 88(245)
syringomyelia 42(256–60)

tactile hallucinations 36(131), 79(84),
   81(123–7), 179[9]
tardive dyskinesia 57(93), 135(236), 161(253),
   183[13]
taste, hallucinations of 129(127)
temporal disturbances 58(121–5), 59(132),
   104(79)
temporal lobe
   functional assessment 125(38), 148(12)
   lesions 65(251)
      epilepsy 81(127)
      non-dominant 101(36), 112(251–5)
tendon reflexes, absent 65(256–60), 161(260)
thalamus, anterior nucleus lesions 136(253)
therapeutic index 55(62)
Thorndike's law of effect 99(11)
thought(s), audible 204[34]
thought blocking 154(126), 204[34]
thought broadcasting 37(168), 85(198),
   106(143)
thyroid function tests 189[19]
time-related disturbances/disorders 58(121–5),
   59(132), 104(79)
torsades de pointes 213[43]
torticollis, spasmodic 136(256–60)
Tourette syndrome 150(44)
toxicity of drugs see adverse drug reactions
Trail Making Test 54(42), 125(37)
transference 38(175–9), 38(190), 61(175–6),
   131(158)

transient ischaemic attacks 187[17]
transitional object 125(47), 157(181–5)
trazodone, adverse effects 34(97), 103(69)
treatment, explaining *19*
tricyclic antidepressants
  adverse reactions 56(82–6), 79(63–7),
    152(68–72)
   in abrupt withdrawal 128(81–5)
  chlorpromazine and 102(51)
trifluoperazine 77(38)
twilight states 82(144)

uncal lesions 65(252)
uraemia 61(180)
urinary infection 186[16]
urine
  drug screen 199[29]
  mid-stream, cultures 200[30]

vascular (multi-infarct) dementia 161(244),
  184[14], 187[17]
vicarious reinforcement 75(12)
visual accommodation, drugs adversely
  affecting 34(94–8)
visual hallucinations 35(110), 59(133),
  60(153), 80(103), 106(130), 129(128),
  153(93)

visual imagery during encoding 30(21),
  123(7)
vitamin B_{12} deficiency 105(102–6), 174[4]
volume of distribution 55(64, 68–70)
voluntary movements, abnormal 135(236–40)

Wechsler's Adult Intelligence Scale–Revised
  54(38), 77(33), 125(36), 148(12)
Wechsler's Memory Scale–Revised 54(46)
weight gain, drug-induced 34(89–93), 79(64)
Wernicke's aphasia 31(48)
Wernicke's encephalopathy 112(256–60),
  176[6]
Wilson's disease 40(216)
Wisconsin Card Sorting Test 54(43), 101(37)
witzelsucht 179[9]
Word Association Technique 123(9)
working alliance 131(156–60)
written examination *3*
  marking system *3*
  outline *5*
  time *3*
  see also extended matching items;
    individual statement questions

zopiclone 101(44)